Want to know how much fat you are carrying around?

READ CHAPTER FOUR

In order to measure your percent of body fat, accurate, low-priced skinfold calipers with instructions for use can be obtained from:

Diet's End
P.O. Box 8009
Prairie Village, Kansas
66208

Enclose $24.95 plus $3.00 shipping and handling for each skinfold caliper ordered.

Published in the United States by Norman Rose

Owing to limitations of space, all acknowledgements for permission to reprint previously published material may be found on pages 342 and 343.

ISBN 0-9631847-1-7

Manufactured in the United States of America

Second Edition

If you have coronary heart disease, diabetes, other health problems or suspected health problems please consult your physician before beginning any weight loss program or undergoing drastic dietary changes.

This book is intended as a helpful tool, not as a substitute for conventional medical therapy.

***

Often times the first symptoms of coronary heart disease is instant death.

Dedicated to all those folks who have fought the fight against fat and failed. May you find your solution in the following pages.

" **A**nd ye shall eat old store, and bring forth the old because of the new."

Leviticus 26:10

have this condition, one which is now known to be perfectly treatable. They, too, can avoid the suffering, incapacitation and all too often lethal consequences of arteriosclerotic disease. Norman Rose has done it and anyone who follows his advice should be able to do it as well.

Author's Note

The basic thrust, drive, foundation and all-encompassing direction of this book is based on the following truth:

Homo Sapiens (you), were not designed to burn liquid vegetable oil, pig fat or beef fat as "the" primary body fuel!

If you are currently cooking for other people, using excessive oils and fats then you are probably contributing to: (a) their slow deterioration in health (b) increased inefficiency, (c) reduced quality of life (d) burgeoning national health care expenses.

Knowing what I know now, I'm sure that I contributed to my father's early death (at 65) by feeding him a diet very heavy in animal fats. He died from gall bladder disease and a diseased heart. His first heart attack occurred when he was just 35 years old and as a result he was never the same. For his first 35 years his light burned brightly then for 30 years it flickered and went out. I believe we were designed to burn brightly our whole life, then flicker momentarily, and go out.

If you insist on eating copious amounts of fat then you should be prepared to endure an inferior quality of life and not just a premature death. You should be prepared to be a burden on the family, the community and the nation.

If you didn't know the down-side of excessive fat consumption then you conducted yourself, as I did, in ignorance.

Chapter 1
Fat and Oil

Until you take the excessive fat and oils out of your diet, you are bound to fail in your attempts to control your weight permanently and to become physically fit.

"All oils are pure 100% fat. All oils contain saturated fat. Fat makes you fat. Therefore, if you are fat, all oils should be your number one enemy. The reason for this is quite simple: oils are sneaky! Animal fat should rank number two because at least you know your enemy." I said this in my first book, "No Fat Please" and it is still true.

Now that we have identified fat people's enemy number one and two let's look at three fundamental truths that have evolved over the last several decades.

Truth Number One

Your brain and stomach don't help much in your weight loss or weight control efforts.

When you substantially reduce the amount of food you consume each day, the stomach becomes convinced that throat has been cut, or at least severely constricted. The message from the stomach to the brain reads something like this:

MEMO
TO: Brain
FROM: Stomach
SUBJECT: Eminent Demise

Throat has repeatedly refused to send down calories sufficient to maintain current weight. Starvation has ensued. Suggest you examine the possibility of famine. Meanwhile, please take action to slow down the burning of existing available fuel in the form of stored body fat. If no action is taken, it is my opinion that death is at hand.

The brain takes immediate action by slowing down the fuel burning process (metabolism) thus:

MEMO

TO: All Cells
FROM: Brain
SUBJECT: More Work On Less Fuel

Effective immediately all fuel allotments are hereby reduced by 10%, however, energy output is expected to remain at current levels. Should calorie shortage continue a further reduction is possible. Keep up the good work. Thanks.

Most dieters are aware of "Plateaus" or "Brick Walls" when weight loss is almost impossible to attain, thanks to a brain that is worried about its continuing source of fuel and survival. In this regard, the brain is a highly developed organ perfectly capable of changing body metabolism based upon input from other body components.

The negative communication from stomach to brain agitates the brain to action.

The principles and techniques in this book will stop negative communications from the stomach to the brain, because the stomach will be full and happy!

<u>Truth Number Two</u>

Most people are not going to easily change their regular established menus, after the diet, with unfamiliar foods.

Many people, invariably, revert back to their regular foods. According to Dr William Castelli, the director of the famous Framingham Heart Study, most Americans eat the same ten meals week in and week out.

Those ten meals, with rare exception, are very high in fat and provide fuel that is easily converted into stored body fat. What follows most diets is almost immediate weight gain even though food volume may not be as large as it was prior to the diet.

Looking back over your lifetime it is very apparent that food as a response to stress was introduced at birth, literally on day "one". You cried and something warm with food in it was stuck in your mouth. It didn't matter what caused the crying, food was the obvious and quick solution. Along through early childhood certain foods and menus became mainstays. During adolescence, menus are most certainly self-modified. Then during young adulthood and cohabitation, foods and menus are seemingly etched in stone, as are your eating habits in response to everyday stress.

Many people who avail themselves to weight loss clinics, diet centers and medically assisted programs of weight control are exposed to proper foods and positive directions for a sensible approach to weight control. However, many participants revert back to the old familiar foods once the direct supervision is removed.

If these foods, menus and eating habits are in fact "etched in stone" then it is very difficult to change them. Where then are we to look for a successful approach to weight control after the diet? Let's look at the next "Truth".

Truth Number Three

When you eat a total of 20 grams of fat each day for women or 30 grams for men, it is difficult to gain weight unless you overdose on sugar and become truly sedentary.

Dr. Dean Ornish in his landmark book "Dr. Dean's Ornish's Program for Reversing Heart Disease" lets us know that the average person needs only 14 grams of fat each day. Unfortunately, the average person eats up to ten times that amount each day, and therein lies the problem.

If the problem is too much fat in the diet then it follows part of the solution is to take the fat out of the traditional daily diet.

Chapter 2

The Bad Effects Of Excessive Fat

Most Americans don't worry about heart disease until after "the big one", as the late Redd Fox would say. Likewise, you probably don't care that 80% of those people with Type II diabetes are overweight which has contributed to the development of the disease. And if I tell you that high dietary fat has been linked to cancer, specifically of the breast, prostate, and colon, your internal response is, "NOT ME". Now that I have given due effort to inform you of the really devastating fat-related diseases that can do you in, I ask that you read the next paragraph with a high degree of interest.

Now this is "THE" paragraph. This paragraph will tell you why you should take the excessive fat out of your diet. It is specifically directed towards you guys who have this big innertube of fat around your midsection and you gals who now wear moomoos, tent-like dresses, and pregnant clothes even though you are not pregnant. DIETARY FAT HAS MADE YOU LOOK AND ACT DIFFERENTLY THAN YOU NORMALLY WOULD LOOK AND ACT. The "LOOK" part is self explanatory. The "ACT" part is not so evident to most people.

Too much body fat lowers your quality of life. The first thing to go is stamina which is defined as resistance to fatigue, illness, and hardship. Recently an NFL football team, in a dietary experiment, raised the level of fat in the team meals. Players were tested for treadmill performance before and after the high-fat regimen. Peak performance took a real drop after the inclusion of high levels of dietary fat. As soon as the fat diet was discontinued, their performance returned to the original levels. I am frequently asked about low fat diets pertaining to teenagers and I respond by addressing improved physical stamina and sports.

Stamina as resistance to illness and disease has been clearly demonstrated in many research projects, the most notable disease being coronary heart disease. High on the list of probabilities are breast cancer in women and prostate cancer in men. Not only should you follow your doctors directions for X-rays and exams, you should also follow common-sense prevention techniques in the form of a low-fat diet.

Stamina, as resistance to hardship, is well understood by most overfat folks. Many people eat when subjected to stress. Usually, the food is high in fat and promptly goes into storage as body fat. More stress, more food, more fat in storage. Pretty soon, all that fat in storage begins to create its own stress. The cycle becomes more treacherous and a person is creating his or her own mental and physical hardships. These hardships are directly caused by excessive dietary fat. A simple way to break this cycle is to lower the dietary fat content to about 10% of total calories. You will find it almost impossible to gain weight on a 10% fat diet!

Finally, current research suggests that 75% of deaths due to heart disease and cancer could be eliminated by two simple prevention efforts. These prevention efforts are, eliminate tobacco and incorporate a proper low fat balanced diet.

Chapter 3
The Balancing Act

Winning the War on Eating Habits

Bad eating habits die hard. Most of us who have poorly balanced diets formed our eating patterns at an early age. After finishing previous diet plans, did you find yourself straying back to the old foods?

Instead of trying in vain to eat new foods, why not find ways of preparing the foods you love in ways that are not fattening? This recipe book contains the secrets of preparing satisfying meals that look, taste, and satisfy the same cravings, yet help your body get back in balance in the mean time.

Why is it so hard for some of us to eat what is good for us? I think it dates to man's prehistory. Early Cro-Magnon babies learned from their parents what was safe to eat by the time they reached the crawling/investigating age. A strange berry or plant could be poisonous, so Cro-Magnon young learned to develop a taste for what their parents gave them at an early age. This act of learning what was safe to eat probably qualifies as a "learned instinct". In other words, some foods are instinctively "good" and others are not acceptable.

We still have this instinct. By the time we learn to crawl, we have formed the tastes and food preferences that we'll have the rest of our lives. It is my personal observation when pre-crawling babies that are purposely exposed to a wide variety of foods they grow up and readily accept and enjoy that same wide variety of food. I'm convinced that early exposure to such foods branded them safe and desirable. Perhaps, the rest of us, with weight problems, had limited exposure to balanced diets. As adults, we intellectually know that the four basic food groups are:

1. Protein
2. Bread
3. Fruits and Vegetables
4. Dairy

but our behaviors insist that the four food groups are:

1. Cheeseburgers and Pizza
2. French Fries and Chips
3. Chocolate
4. Cakes and Sweets

If this is the way your instincts behave, you face two problems getting your diet balanced. First the variety of foods you consume will be severely limited. For instance, in your last diet program, did you find yourself counting as vegetables the pickles, tomatoes, lettuce, and mayonnaise that you find on a cheeseburger? Or the mushrooms and peppers on your pizza? We'll deal with this problem in another chapter.

THE MAJOR problem of an instinctively unbalanced diet is the excessive fat content. In order to overcome this fat obstacle you must learn to purchase and prepare fat-free foods that fit into your group of acceptable foods.

Getting back on balance is easier if we don't try to fight our food instincts head on, but gently nudge them in the right direction. This can be done by eating many of the same foods you enjoyed before, but prepared in ways that restrict dietary fat.

Four Requirements for Fat Reduction

The recipes included in this book will seek to bring about weight loss by concentrating on four basic requirements. I want you to think of them just as you would the four basic food groups:

1. Protein
2. Fat
3. Carbohydrates
4. Physical Exercise

Now let's explore these requirements.

Protein Requirements

The average adult needs no more than two ounces of protein a day. Protein is required to build muscles, repair damaged tissue, and produce mother's milk.

Does two ounces sound small? I assure you, the quarter-pound cheeseburger you wolfed down for a snack contains at least half the protein your body needs for the whole day. (and any fried meat is overloaded with fat that you don't need at all.) ONLY if you are a serious body builder trying to look like Arnold Schwarzenegger, AND you happen to be pregnant, AND you have the worst cold of your life, AND you have your arm broken in three places, AND you are breast feeding twins - then and only then - will I concede that you probably require more than two ounces of protein a day.

All protein you consume in excess is converted by the body to fuel. Unfortunately, protein is a very inefficient fuel resulting in ammonia as a byproduct. Ammonia is toxic and must be flushed rapidly from the body.

Why then, you ask, have highly-publicized weight-loss programs you've tried centered on high protein consumption? These programs get quick results, which our impatient "I want it now" society teaches us to look for. High protein diets at best result in temporary weight loss and at worst teach your body how to gain weight faster.

High-protein/low-calorie diets APPEAR to result in weight loss, but the truth is that high-protein diets are not efficient in eliminating fatty weight: much of the weight loss experienced is water and muscle.

I hope you will underline or circle this next sentence: High-protein/low-calorie diets cause the body to GAIN WEIGHT FASTER THAN EVER as soon as the diet is over.

Why is this true? Several reasons. We've stated that excess protein results in overproduction of ammonia, which the body must rapidly flush away to survive. Huge amounts of protein result in huge amounts of ammonia that must be flushed out. This flushing action depletes the body of water and gives a false sense of losing weight. A small number of people get very ill from such diets because their kidneys just can't keep up.

Water is very heavy. Try lifting a five-gallon bucket of water and you'll see what I mean. One pint of water weighs a little more than one pound. A small increase in the rate of water eliminated by the body will show up as weight loss. But this is not the weight loss you really want and need! Once you stop the high-protein diet and the stress of excessive ammonia is removed from your kidneys, the body will rapidly seek to build back its water supply, gaining back every ounce of water it lost.

Even more insidious is the devastating muscle loss that high-protein/low-calorie diets wreak on the body. These diet plans typically are low in carbohydrates, the foodstuff that is readily converted into glucose (blood sugar). Without carbohydrates to draw from, the body's response is to convert protein into glucose. If the amount of protein absorbed from the diet plan proves insufficient to supply the needed quantity of glucose, then the body simply devours its own muscles in order to create adequate levels of blood sugar or glucose.

This is truly a double disaster. As you'll learn elsewhere in this book, only muscles can burn fat. If you lose muscle mass, you reduce your ability to burn dietary fat. To your horror, you'll discover that you will gain weight easier and faster after your high-protein/low-calorie diet is over.

On a typical high protein diet, only a fraction of the apparent weight loss is really due to decreased fat. For every pound of fat lost, another pound of muscle is lost, and more than a pound of water is lost. Let's say for sake of argument that a friend of yours has just lost 32 pounds on a high-protein/low-calorie diet. In reality, he has lost:

10 pounds fat
10 pounds muscle
<u>12 pounds water</u>
32 pounds total weight loss

As soon as your friend stops this high-protein/low-calorie diet, he will rapidly put back on 12 pounds of water weight. With a reduced ability to burn dietary fat, your friend will find that his body will acquire fat quicker than it did before the diet. Unless your friend has embarked upon a sincere exercise program (and most of us don't), fat will replace the lost muscle mass as well. How does your friend react? He goes back on the high-protein/low-calorie diet he thought was so successful, and loses even more muscle mass, which of course accelerates even further how fast his body puts on fat. Is it any wonder people get discouraged and say, "I simply cannot lose weight"?

We can all conjure up images of starving people appearing as only skin and bone. Their muscle protein has been converted into glucose so that their brain could survive. The brain is a glucose glutton, using more than 60 times as much as a resting muscle of equal weight. Starving people may pass out because the brain can't get enough glucose.

Fat requirements

Fat is used almost exclusively for fuel to make the muscles go. Believe it or not, vegetable oil which is almost pure fat, burns quite well in a diesel motor, delivering steady and prolonged energy to the drive train. In a similar way, fat provides prolonged energy to your body.

The average person wishing to lose weight should strive to eliminate added fat from his diet. Your minimum daily requirement of fat is 14 grams (about 1/2 ounce), but don't worry about not getting it. In our society that is practically impossible. With all the oils used in prepared foods, the average person consumes ten times the daily fat requirement without trying. That's why the recipes in this book include no added fat or fatty food ingredients.

Our prehistoric ancestors couldn't always count on a meal three times a day, and sources of dietary fat were harder to find. Because our bodies needed a reliable constant source of energy, we evolved to become very efficient at fat storage. Our bodies learned to store fat to use as energy during times when food was hard to find. The easy storage and withdrawal of fat has allowed mankind to survive. Forty thousand years later, our bodies have not yet evolved to cope with the high fat availability in today's food.

Your body's fat reserve is a lot like a bank account, that accepts deposits and withdrawals. If you are consuming 150 grams of fat each day and are neither gaining nor losing weight, it is safe to assume that you are using up 150 grams of fat each day. If tomorrow you consume only 20 grams of fat, your body will withdraw 130 grams from reserve to meet its current 150 grams daily "expenditure." This is in fact a fat loss of 130 grams a day, or about 2 pounds of fat loss a week. The recipes in this book will help keep your fat intake as low as possible, encouraging your body to tap into its fat reserve for its energy needs.

Carbohydrate Requirements

For steady, prolonged physical activities, fat provides most of the fuel. But for explosive bursts of physical activities, carbohydrates are the principle source of energy. In the Midwest, grain silos, occasionally, explode with amazing force. Carbohydrates in the form of wheat dust can be as explosive as dynamite when accidentally ignited in a grain storage facility. Your body uses carbohydrates in much the same way.

If you get your 2 ounce daily requirement of protein and your 14 gram (1/2 ounce) daily requirement of fat, then the rest of your energy requirements should come from carbohydrates. Good sources of carbohydrates are bread, potatoes, rice, corn, pasta, and beans.

Interestingly, beans when combined with grains, also form an excellent source of protein. In some countries beans and rice, or bean tacos almost completely replace meat as a source of protein. Your body readily converts carbohydrates into glucose, which is in turn used as fuel for the muscles and brain.

Physical Activity Requirement

The only way that fat is removed from the body is when it is needed as fuel for muscles. Muscles burn fat! In order to become an efficient fat burner, you must increase your muscle mass, especially those big muscles located in your calves, thighs, and buttocks. These muscles are best developed by simple, steady walking on a daily basis.

A regular walking routine should be your biggest priority. I don't mean speed walking and I don't mean a leisurely la-dee-dah walk, but rather a steady walk. (About the speed you'd use walking to the next gas station after having run out of gas.) Your walk should last for at least 20 minutes at a time, and if possible you should walk 5 or 6 days a week.

An important note: don't count the time you are on your feet in the course of your regular daily routine as exercise. You need to INCREASE the level of your exercise above and beyond what your body receives in a normal day.

If you want to build muscle mass and your fat-burning ability more rapidly, walk longer, not faster. Other activities such as tennis, golf, baseball, and swimming should be considered as fun and games, and NOT part of your minimum physical activity requirement.

Some people's minds are like concrete, all mixed up and permanently set.

Anonymous

Chapter 4

The Importance of Body Composition and Percent of Body Fat*

In recent years, the measurement of percent of body fat has become widely used and recommended as one of the indicators of fitness. By monitoring percent of body fat and weight regularly, there are many things a person can learn about their fitness and any changes in fitness as time progresses, that cannot be learned by weighing with a scale alone. Later in this section I will tell you how to measure percent of body fat, but first I will explain it and tell about the many benefits obtained by monitoring body fat.

Perhaps the most important single thing the monitoring of percent of body fat will do is determine changes in muscle tissue over time. By knowing percent of body fat, the percent of muscle, bone, organs, etc. can also be determined. For example, if a person has 20 percent body fat and weighs 135 pounds, then 27 pounds of this is fat. Everything else, which is sometimes referred to as the "lean mass" is 80 percent of their weight or 108 pounds. Of this lean mass, the component that can change the most is muscle tissue. Therefore, if a person monitors their change in percent of body fat and weight, they can also determine their change in muscle tissue. Muscle tissue can increase or decrease depending on a persons diet, activities, exercise, and lifestyle.

Recent research has shown several interesting things about body composition and muscle tissue. One major study has shown that the typical American loses muscle tissue and

* By Wallace C. Donohue with permission

gains fat steadily from about age 20 on. The study shows that even people of standard weight, who maintain their same weight as they grow older, still gain fat and lose muscle tissue. A study by Brozek and Keys of a large group of men showed the following changes in percent of fat with age of people of standard weight. That is, people who maintained their correct weight per height-weight charts.

Age	20	25	30	35	40	45	50	55
% Body fat	10.3	13.4	16.2	18.6	20.7	22.5	23.9	25.0

What this shows is that a person who weighs, for example, 160 pounds at age 20 has 16 pounds of fat (10.3 percent) and 144 pounds of everything else (bones, muscle, organs, etc.). But at age 55, this same person who still weighs 160 pounds has 40 pounds of fat (25 percent) and 120 pounds of everything else. Since muscle tissue is the component of the "lean mass" that changes the most, this means that from age 20 to age 55, this person has lost 24 pounds of muscle tissue and replaced it with a gain of 24 pounds of fat. Even though this person weighs the same at 55 as he did at 20, his body has deteriorated substantially. The example is given for a man, but exactly the same thing happens to women.

This deterioration did not have to happen to this person. It is due to the typical American lifestyle. It has been shown that those who exercise regularly, along with a proper diet, do not lose muscle tissue or gain fat. In fact, even at age 50 and above, it is possible to build muscle tissue back up and regain the correct balance between muscle, fat, and weight. All that is necessary is the proper exercise and diet program.

It is important to note that the deterioration starts early. Even by the age of 25, the typical American has lost 3 percent of their total body weight in muscle tissue and replaced it with a corresponding increase in the percent of body fat. And this is just for those who maintain their correct weight. For those whose weight increase, the situation is worse because almost all of the weight increase is fat. If a person monitors their percent of body fat regularly, they can detect muscle loss early on and take corrective action before serious changes take place.

Another very important use of the percent of body fat measurements is to monitor the effect of diet and/or exercise on muscle tissue and fat. For example, research has shown that when a person goes on a typical fad diet, with little exercise, they lose as much or more muscle tissue than fat. (Scales will not tell a person this is happening, but measuring the percent of body fat regularly will.) Then, if this person goes off the diet and gains the weight back, they gain more fat back than they lost and less muscle tissue than they lost. The result is that they have more fat and less muscle tissue than before the down-up cycle and are worse off than before the diet. Again, measuring the percent of body fat will show this whereas scales will not.

Of course, the way to reduce properly is through lots of exercise combined with a proper well-balanced diet. In this way it is possible for a person to actually gain muscle tissue while losing fat. Measuring the percent of body fat regularly will determine the effectiveness of the exercise-diet program being used.

There are many other things measuring the percent of body fat can show. For example, a person who is much too lean, particularly women, may not realize this and the scales will not tell them. There are studies which indicate it is harmful for women to drop below 10 to 12 percent body fat. And, of course, we all know the problem of Anorexic girls and women who did not realize, or refuse to believe, they are much too lean. Regular monitoring of the percent of body fat will show graphically and accurately that they are too lean and are also losing muscle and organ tissue with their inadequate nutrition intake. Positive proof of this through the percent of body fat measurements might help convince them that they need a better diet, higher in calories and nutrition.

Another use for the percent of body fat measurements concerns a much more common situation. This is the person who is the correct weight according to a height-weight chart or even underweight according to these charts. They may also look reasonably fit when they look in a mirror and may think they are just fine. And yet, if they measure their percent of body fat they may find they have too much fat. Their small, under-developed, probably little-used muscles account for their light weight. The percent of body fat measurements will show them they are over fat and under muscled and they will realize they need to go on an exercise program to replace fat with muscle.

And yet another possibility is a very strong, muscular, athletic person. They may have a weight considerably above what a height-weight chart would say they should have. If they believe the chart they may think they have to lose weight. This person might actually be very lean and if they were to go on a diet and lose weight almost all the loss would be muscle tissue. Measuring the percent of body fat would reveal this situation and show the person they were lean and that the extra weight was muscle and possibly even stronger bones which have a higher density. A scale cannot give this information. Only the percent of body fat measurements will show this.

A typical situation that exists when someone starts on a good exercise program combined with proper nutrition is that they find their weight is not changing even after several months. They may get discouraged and give it up, thinking their new regimen is not doing them any good. However, if they measured their percent of body fat regularly they would find they were replacing fat with muscle and, in fact, benefiting themselves greatly. Thus, rather than becoming discouraged, they would be encouraged to continue.

Now that the importance of the percent of body fat measurements has been explained, we come to the question of how to measure it. There are two primary methods in use today. One is underwater weighing and the other is Skinfold Caliper measurements. Both are accurate. Underwater weighing tends to be more accurate than Skinfold Calipers for people above 40 percent body fat. For people in the 15 to 40 percent range, Skinfold Calipers and underwater weighing are about equal in accuracy. For people less than 15 percent body fat, underwater weighing becomes progressively less accurate and can be seriously in error for very lean people. Skinfold Calipers are the most accurate method for people below 15 percent body fat. There are several other methods such as circumference measurements, but none are accurate and only provide an approximation.

Underwater weighing is impractical for most people and is generally only used in large facilities such as schools and hospitals. Skinfold Calipers are then the obvious answer for most applications. They are accurate and easy to use and can also be used in the home.

What is the correct or ideal percent of body fat? This is perhaps the most difficult question to answer. Not all people have the same ideal percent of body fat. It varies with age and sex, and one person might be better at a higher or lower percent of body fat than another person of the same age and sex. And the desirable body fat of athletes can vary depending on the sport. For example, swimmers seem to perform at a higher percent of body fat than runners. But, some general guidelines and ranges can be given that are applicable to the vast majority.

For men up to about age 30, 9 to 15 percent is good. From age 30 to 50, 11 to 17 percent is a good range and from age 50 and up, 12 to 19 percent. A person should try to stay below the upper limits given and a person at the lower limit would be described as lean.

For women, the range up to age 30 is 14 to 21 percent, from 30 to 50, 15 to 23 percent, and from 50 up it is 16 to 25 percent. Again, it is desirable to be below the upper limit, and a woman near the lower limit would be lean.

The percent of body fat obtained by underwater weighing or skinfold calipers includes total body fat, not just that under the skin. In addition to the fat under the skin all people have internal fat, around organs, etc. A certain amount of fat is necessary for health and body functioning, sometimes referred to as essential fat. Many people, particularly women, try to get too lean. It is generally agreed that this is not healthy, and, in many cases can actually cause harm. Women should not try to get below the minimums given above.

It should be noted that the ranges given above are not the averages for the U.S. population, but are the desirable ranges. The actual averages for the population as a whole are much higher because of the large number of people with the percent of body fat well above the upper limit of the desirable ranges.

Acceptably accurate, low priced Skinfold Calipers with instructions for use can be obtained from:

Diets End
P.O. Box 8009
Shawnee Mission, KS 66208

Enclose $24.95 plus $3.00 shipping and handling for each Skinfold Caliper ordered.

TO CALCULATE YOUR DESIRED WEIGHT

Example:

Pat weighs 150 lbs., is over-fat with a percent body-fat content of 33% and desires a content of 25%. What will the new weight figure be?

First:
Compute your "Lean Mass"
Line "A" Current weight = 150 lbs.
Line "B" Current % Body Fat = 33%

Total Body Fat = Line "A" multiplied by line "B" with a decimal point in front of the line "B" figure.

Line "C" 150 x .33 = 50 lbs.

Line "A" minus line "C" equals lean mass:
150 - 50 = 100 lbs.

Line "D" Pat's lean mass = 100 lbs.

Second:
Multiply your lean mass from line "D" by the multiplication factor from column "B". This will give you your new desired weight.

This side is for your personal computations.

A. Current weight _____ lbs.

B. Current % body fat _____ %

Total body fat = Line "A" Multiplied by line "B" with a decimal point in front of the line "B" figure.

C. ____ X .____ = ____ lbs.

Line "A" ____ minus Line "C" ___ = ___ lbs.

Your lean mass = ___ lbs.
Lean mass multiplied by column "B" = Desired Weight

Column "A" Desired Percentage of Body Fat	Column "B" Multiplication Factor
25% =	1.330
24% =	1.315
23% =	1.298
22% =	1.282
21% =	1.265
20% =	1.250
19% =	1.234
18% =	1.219
17% =	1.204
16% =	1.190
15% =	1.176

"It was a pleasant morning in September 1990. I had just completed a "routine" treadmill. The cardiologist called me into his office and stated matter of factly, "You are a walking time bomb. I would like you to check into the hospital this afternoon." Two days later the surgeon opened my chest and stitched in by passes to six clogged arteries.

That got my attention. Before my surgery my nutrition motto was "Life is uncertain... eat dessert first." and if I got the urge to exercise I would lay down until it went away. Suddenly I became highly motivated to learn what food to put into my body to keep my arteries clear. I suddenly "found the time" to exercise and I devoured every book I could find on exercise, nutrition and stress management.

Within a few weeks I became more energetic, endurance increased, I lost several pounds and my mental capacity even seemed sharper. At 60 years of age I felt 25 years younger. **I became hooked on exercise and proper nutrition!**

In July 1992 I retired from 42 years of banking to open the *Vital Life Center* which is dedicated to my new passion... helping people to stay well and feel great. I discovered Norm's first book, **NO FAT PLEASE**, while on vacation in Branson, MO and I am making it "required reading" for my clients. It is chocked full of great recipes and common sense!"

Gene Millen, President
Vital Life Center
3184 Collins Drive
Merced, CA 95340

Chapter 5

Good Calories, Bad Calories, Fat and the Menu

I personally don't think in terms of calories. I always think in terms of how many grams of fat per serving. My basic "fat" rule is: NO MORE THAN 1 GRAM OF FAT PER SERVING.

The only exception to this rule is meat, poultry, fish, and meat substitutes. For these items I try to observe the "1 gram of fat per ounce" rule. This gives me my choice of:

(a) Breast of chicken
(b) Breast of turkey
(c) Venison
(b) Buffalo
(e) Low fat fish
(b) Harvest Burgers®

I like beef, so occasionally I do indulge. However, beef sirloin (lean only, broiled) measures in at about 2.4 grams of fat per ounces, which means that a 6 ounce cut would contain about 14.4 grams of fat. As you will see later in this chapter, is you restrict your "filet" choices to chicken, turkey, venison, buffalo, fish, or Harvest Burgers®, then your entire days consumption of fat is just 14.6 grams.

I like my "fat" rule because it is so simple. When I look at a label I look for "Fat" and then the amount. If it says 1 gram or less, then it fits into the plan. If it says 2 grams or more, I put it down very quickly and go on about my business. As you can see all I need to be able to read is the word "Fat" and understand the mathematics of the number "1", which is:

Fat = 1 gram = OK

Fat = 2 grams = DON'T BUY

This means I don't buy shortening, lard, cooking oil, butter, margarine, peanut butter, nuts, potato chips, corn chips, and other products that contain more than 1 gram of fat per serving. When adhering to this rule I simply can't gain weight, and yet I eat a lot of really great food and I never feel deprived.

But for those of you who feel compelled to count calories you should know that all calories are not created equal, and you will have to learn the difference between "fat" calories and "carbohydrate" or "protein" calories. Current research at Cornell University indicates that what you eat (not necessarily how much) is the main factor behind weight control.

In the longest controlled human-feeding study ever undertaken, Cornell University nutritionists have found that people on low-fat diets lose weight. What's more, people on low-fat diets continue to lose weight for months without suffering hunger pangs, craving foods, or becoming depressed.

In the 22-week study, 13 women whose average age was 34 were asked to eat a carefully controlled regular- or low-fat laboratory diet, and their food intake and weight loss were monitored. The scientists found that the women on low-fat diets steadily lost weight--about one-half pound per week.

David Levitsky, professor of nutrition and of psychology at Cornell University, published results of the study in the May 1991, issue of the American Journal of Clinical Nutrition. Co-authors are lecturer Anne Kendall-Casela and senior research associate and adjunct professor of psychology Barbara J. Strupp, both of Cornell.

Previous studies have strongly suggested when dieters reduce their carbohydrates, or substitute artificial sweeteners for sugar, they fully compensate for these calorie deficits by eating more from other food groups, Levitsky explained.

"In our studies on low-fat diets, though, there's no evidence that less fat in the diet results in a person feeling more hungry, having food cravings or compensating for the calorie deficit. Dieters can still eat ice cream, cookies and pizza--just low-fat versions," said Levitsky.

The Cornell University low fat diet allowed approximately 40-50 grams of fat per day.

Incidentally, every nutritionist in the world agrees on the issue of a low fat diet.

As to what is the difference between a "fat" calorie and a "carbohydrate" or "protein" calorie, it is this: during digestion the body uses much more energy in converting excess protein or carbohydrates into fat for storage. For example, if you eat 100 calories of carbohydrates that are not needed, then your body burns up about 25 of those calories when converting them to body fat, whereas for each 100 calories of excess fat eaten, 97 are turned into body fat. This is an enormous difference and it is half of the solution that allows you to provide a 1600 calorie diet that provides volume, texture, flavor, and the perception of old fashioned "regular" food. The other half of the solution is the fact that 1 gram of fat equals 9 calories whereas 1 gram of carbohydrate or protein equals just 4 calories. Fat is a very dense source of energy and if you take from the diet 10 grams of fat at 90 calories and replace it with 22.5 grams of carbohydrates at 90 calories, I think you can see that you would eat over twice as much (by weight). This fact makes for a happy stomach when you present the following 1600 calorie "diet" to a husky 200-pound fellow.

Breakfast
3 waffles
1 cup fresh strawberries, sliced
4 tablespoons maple flavored syrup
coffee or tea

Lunch
Sweet & sour chicken on rice
Fresh sliced vegetables
Diet cola, coffee, tea, or water

Dinner (supper)
6 ounce bacon-wrapped filet
Baked potato, sour cream and butter sauce
Vegetable/shrimp kabob with butter sauce
2 large feather-light biscuits

For gals looking for a 1300 calorie menu, just remove 1 waffle, 1/2 baked potato, and one biscuit.

Let's itemize and analyze this menu and understand that purchasing and preparation are keenly important in controlling the amount of fat in any diet. If you buy wrong, you can't possibly eat right.

	Grams of Fat	Calories
Breakfast		
3 Waffles (frozen, fat free)	1	240
4 Tablespoons of lite butter flavored syrup	0	100
1 Cup of fresh strawberries, sliced	0	45
Coffee/Tea, plain or artificial sweetener	0	0
Total	1	385

	Grams of Fat	Calories
Lunch		
Sweet & sour chicken	2	140
Rice (1 cup)	0	225
Fresh sliced peppers, carrots, and celery	0	30
Diet cola, unsweetened tea, water,		
or coffee (no cream)	0	6
Total	2	401
Dinner		
1 baked potato (8 ounces)	0	220
1 ounce "lite" sour cream	2	30
1 strip turkey bacon	2	25
6-ounce mesquite broiled filet	6.6	318
Vegetable/shrimp kabob	.5	40
Butter sauce	0	0
2 big biscuits	1.5	200
Total fat	12.6	
Minus fat loss during cooking	-1.0	
Totals	11.6	833

Analysis

	Fat Content	Total Calories
Breakfast	1 gram	385
Lunch	2 grams	401
Dinner	11.6 grams	833
Totals	14.6 grams	1619

Calories from fat =   131.4
Percent of calories from fat =   8.1%
Grams of saturated fat =   7.55
Percent of calories from saturated fat =   4.1%
Total cholesterol =   160.6 MG
(with buffalo filet)

Once you get the hang of it, you will find that
scrambled eggs (fat-free substitute), bacon, hash

browns, and biscuits also fit into your breakfast menu. And how about sticky buns, Irish soda bread toast and jam, creamy oatmeal and scones, fresh fruit, cold cereals, bagels and "cream cheese", along with steak and gravy over feather lite biscuits. These are just some possible breakfast items. I'm sure whatever your favorite item is, it can probably be purchased and prepared fat free.

The selected lunch menu here was, in fact, left over from the night before. I find it is an easy solution to the problem of what to have for lunch. Just prepare enough the night before so as to allow for the number of lunches you'll need tomorrow. Zap it in the microwave at work. Lunch, you'll discover, could have been a chicken and green chile burrito, cold sandwich, hot sandwich, or any evening entree you prepare.

The dinner (supper here in the midwest) menu has an almost unlimited number of possible combinations. If you are trying to eliminate cholesterol, your filet would be a cholesterol free Midland Harvest Burger®. You would replace the shrimp with scallops and probably not eat the turkey bacon. If you crave red meat, I know you'll love farm raised venison or buffalo. I'll tell you later in chapters 10 and 11 where and how to purchase these items that are so low in fat and cholesterol. Of course chicken, turkey, and fish wrapped in bacon and grilled over a mesquite fire are always good. When you get to the point where you can afford to eat another 300 calories, just throw in a slab of pie or a slice of cake - just make sure they are FAT FREE.

Cooking and preparing this same menu the old fashioned American way would have resulted in an extra 1,614 calories bringing the daily total to 3,233. The fat content likewise shoots up like a sky rocket adding an extra 126.8 grams of fat for a total fat content of 141.4 grams. The "American" way, provides 39.3% of your daily calories from fat, which puts many people in the coronary intensive care unit of the local hospital.

Any discussion of bad calories would be lacking without the inclusion of alcohol calories.

A good wine with good food can be soul satisfying. A cold glass of beer on a hot summer day can be a welcomed thirst-quencher. The New Testament exhorts us to "use a little wine for the stomach's sake and thine often infirmities"... I Timothy 5:12. If you look for justification for the use of alcohol I'm sure you can find it, however you should know a few pertinent facts about alcohol calories.

According to Paolo M. Suter, M.D. (Ethanol and Fat Storage - Suter et at, New England Journal of Medicine, Vol. 326, No. 14, April 9, 1992) ALCOHOL SIGNIFICANTLY SLOWS THE BURNING OF FAT IN YOUR BODY. Three ounces of alcohol in a 24 hour period will reduce the amount of fat burned by about 50 grams. This equates to about 3/4 pound of fat placed in storage for each 7 day fishing trip with the beer drinking buddies.

Another way to state the results of this study would be to say that 3 ounces of alcohol will reduce the number of calories burned by about 1/3 in a given day.

Apparently the body first burns the alcohol, then carbohydrates and protein and lastly the body burns some fat and puts the rest in storage.

If you want to be a social drinker, you should attempt to substitute the alcohol calories for fat calories. Although you may be able to control your weight this way your body-fat content will probably increase and tend to turn you into a jelly fish.

The one word summarizing alcohol consumption is moderation.

Chapter 6

So You Have High Blood Cholesterol

Medical information in this chapter has been provided by the U.S. Department of Health and Human Services, Public Health Service, National Institute of Health.

I have included this chapter in order to help disseminate the story of blood cholesterol and the devastating effects of elevated levels upon our society and the very fabric of our democratic existence.

As health care expenditures continue to sky rocket, I question how long, we as a nation, can sustain our economic growth pattern of the past with the attendant high quality-of-life standards.

It has been stated recently that 75% of deaths due to heart disease and cancer could be eliminated by the mastering of two problems. Those two problems are tobacco and diet.

Anyone can develop high blood cholesterol regardless of age, sex, race, or ethnic background. But, because there are no warning symptoms or signs, you are likely to be surprised at such a diagnosis. Don't be alarmed, but do take it seriously. Like high blood pressure, most people are unaware that their blood cholesterol levels are high until they learn it from their doctor. And, like high blood pressure, it is a potential threat to your health that you can do something about.

If you have just learned that you have high blood cholesterol, there are some important facts you need to know to protect your health. First, you need to find out what high blood cholesterol is, how high your level is, and what you can do to lower it. Then prepare to make some changes. Although these changes will depend on many factors considered by your doctor, modifying your diet is the preferred way to lower blood cholesterol.

This chapter will answer many of the questions you may have about your blood cholesterol level. The glossary will help you become familiar with the terms used in this chapter and in other information about cholesterol.

High blood cholesterol is one of the three major risk factors for coronary heart disease (cigarette smoking and high blood pressure are the other two). In other words, high blood cholesterol can significantly increase your risk of developing heart disease. Fortunately, all three risk factors are "modifiable"; that is, you can do something about them. You can take steps to lower your cholesterol level and thus lower your risk for coronary heart disease.

High blood cholesterol occurs when there is too much cholesterol in your blood. Your cholesterol level is determined partly by your genetic makeup and the saturated fat and cholesterol in the foods you eat. Even if you didn't eat any cholesterol, your body would manufacture enough for its needs.

The risk of developing coronary heart disease increases as your blood cholesterol level rises. This is why it is so important that you have your blood cholesterol level measured. Currently, more than half of all adult Americans have blood cholesterol levels of 200 mg/dl or greater, which places them at an increased risk for coronary heart disease. Approximately 25 percent of the adult population 20 years of age or older has blood cholesterol levels that are considered "high", that is, 240 mg/dl greater.

Your doctor will measure your level with a blood sample taken from your finger or your arm and will confirm this result with a second test if it is greater than 200 mg/dl. The following table can help you see how the results of your total blood cholesterol tests relate to your risk of developing coronary heart disease.

Desirable Blood Cholesterol	Borderline-High Blood Cholesterol	High Blood Cholesterol
Less than 200 mg/dl	200 to 239 mg/dl	240 mg/dl and above

Note: These categories apply to anyone 20 years of age or older.

A blood cholesterol level of 240 mg/dl or greater is considered "high" blood cholesterol. But any level above 200 mg/dl, even in the "borderline-high" category, increases your risk for heart disease. If your blood cholesterol is 240 mg/dl or greater, you have more than twice the risk of someone whose cholesterol is 200 mg/dl, and you need medical attention and further testing.

When your high blood cholesterol level is combined with another major risk factor (either high blood pressure or cigarette smoking), your risk for coronary heart disease increases even further. For example, if your cholesterol level is in the "high" category and you have high blood pressure, your risk for coronary heart disease increases six times. If you also smoke, your risk increases more than 20-fold. Other factors that increase your risk for coronary heart disease include a family history of coronary heart disease before the age of 55, diabetes, vascular (blood vessel) disease, obesity, and being male. Whether your total blood cholesterol is in the "borderline-high" category or "high" category, you should make some changes in your diet to lower your level. More specifically, if your level is in the "borderline-high" category and you have coronary heart disease or two other risk factors for coronary heart disease or is in the "high" category, your physician will prescribe more aggressive treatment and follow your cholesterol levels more closely. If your cholesterol level is desirable, you should have your level checked again in 5 years and take steps to prevent it from rising.

Risk Factors For Coronary Heart Disease
High blood cholesterol
High blood pressure
Cigarette smoking
Family history of coronary heart
  disease before the age of 55
Diabetes
Vascular disease
Obesity
Being male

Most coronary heart disease is caused by atherosclerosis, which occurs when cholesterol, fat, and other substances build up in the walls of the arteries that supply blood to the heart. These deposits narrow the arteries and can slow or block the flow of blood. Among many things, blood carries a constant supply of oxygen to the heart. Without oxygen, heart muscle weakens, resulting in chest pain (angina), a heart attack (myocardial infarction), or even death. Atherosclerosis is a slow progressive disease that may start very early in life, yet might not produce symptoms for many years.

Lowering your high blood cholesterol level will slow fatty buildup in the walls of the arteries and reduce your risk of a heart attack and death caused by a heart attack. In fact, some studies have shown that, in adults with "high" blood cholesterol levels, for each 1 percent reduction in total cholesterol levels, there is a 2 percent reduction in the number of heart attacks. In other words, if your reduce your cholesterol level 15 percent, your risk of coronary heart disease could drop by 30 percent.

- Diet: Among the factors you can do something about, diet has the largest effect on your blood cholesterol level. <u>Saturated fat raises your blood cholesterol level more than anything else you eat</u>. Dietary cholesterol also increases your blood cholesterol level. If you have high blood cholesterol, changing your diet will be a very important step to lower it.

- Weight: Being overweight may also increase your blood cholesterol level. Most overweight patients with high levels of cholesterol can help lower their levels by weight reduction.

- Physical activity/exercise: Although it is not clear whether physical activity can prevent atheroslerosis, regular exercise may help you control weight, lower your blood pressure, and increase your level of HDL-cholesterol, the "good" type of blood cholesterol.

- Genetic factors: Genetic factors play a major role in determining your blood cholesterol level and can determine your ability to lower your level by diet. A small number of people have an inherited tendency to have a high blood cholesterol level. If you have a genetic disorder contributing to a high blood cholesterol level, then your parents, children, brothers, and sisters should also have their blood cholesterol levels measured.

- Sex/age: Coronary heart disease is the leading cause of death and disability for both men and women in the United States.

Estimates are that 1 out of 5 men and 1 out of 17 women will have symptoms of heart disease before the age of 60. This means that men have two to three times the risk of developing heart disease as women. However, in women as in men, cholesterol levels are predictive of coronary heart disease.

In the United States, blood cholesterol levels in men and women start to rise at about age 20. Women's blood cholesterol levels prior to menopause (45-60 years) are lower than those of men of the same age. After menopause, however, the cholesterol level of women usually increases to a level higher than that of men. In men, blood cholesterol levels off around age 50 and the average blood cholesterol level declines slightly after age 50. Since the risk of coronary heart disease is especially high in the later decades of life, reducing blood cholesterol levels may be important in the elderly.

In addition, oral contraceptives and pregnancy can increase blood cholesterol levels in some women. For pregnant women, blood cholesterol levels should return to normal 20 weeks after delivery.

- Alcohol: You may have heard that modest amounts of alcohol can improve your cholesterol profile by increasing your HDL-cholesterol level. However, it is not known whether the higher level produced by alcohol protects against coronary heart disease. With this in mind and because drinking can have serious adverse effects, alcohol is not recommended in the prevention of coronary heart disease.

- Stress: Although stress has been reported to raise blood cholesterol levels, there may be other explanations for this effect. For example, during periods of stress, people may eat more foods that are high in saturated fat and cholesterol, which may increase their blood cholesterol levels - rather than the stress itself.

While all of these factors can influence your blood cholesterol level, clearly you can do something about a number of them. In fact, most people are able to lower their blood cholesterol levels with diet alone.

What is Blood Cholesterol?

Cholesterol is an odorless, soft, waxy substance. Your body needs cholesterol to function normally (for example, as a component of cell membranes and for the production of many hormones, vitamin D, and bile acids - which are important for the absorption of fat). Cholesterol is present in all parts of the body, including the brain and nervous system, muscle, skin, liver, intestines, heart, skeleton, etc.

The cholesterol level of your blood is affected by:

- The cholesterol your body produces
- The saturated fat and cholesterol in your diet

Your blood cholesterol level is affected not only by the saturated fat and cholesterol in your diet, but also by the cholesterol your body produces. As a matter of fact, your body produces all the cholesterol it needs, and the saturated fat and cholesterol in your diet only serve to increase your blood cholesterol level.

Cholesterol travels in the blood in packages called lipoproteins. All lipoproteins are formed in the liver and carry cholesterol through the body.

Blood cholesterol packaged in low density lipoproteins (LDLs) is transported from the liver to other parts of the body where it can be used. LDLs carry most of the cholesterol in the blood, and if not removed from the blood, cholesterol and fat can build up in the arteries contributing to atherosclerosis. This is why LDL-cholesterol is often called "bad cholesterol".

Cholesterol is also packaged in high density lipoproteins (HDLs). HDLs carry cholesterol back to the liver for processing or removal from the body. HDLs therefore help remove cholesterol from the blood, preventing the accumulation of cholesterol in the walls of the arteries. Thus they are often referred to as "good cholesterol".

If your total cholesterol level is either in the "high" category or in the "borderline-high" category and you have coronary heart disease or two other risk factors for coronary heart disease, your doctor will want a more complete "cholesterol profile" that includes LDL-cholesterol, HDL-cholesterol levels, and triglyceride levels. A blood test provides this information: you will have to fast for 12 hours prior to the test. (You may notice that your LDL- and HDL-cholesterol levels do not add up to your total blood cholesterol level. LDLs usually carry about 60-70 percent and HDLs about 25 percent of the total cholesterol in your blood. Other lipoproteins carry the rest.)

Some laboratories may calculate your cholesterol ratio. This measurement is actually just your total cholesterol or LDL-cholesterol divided by your HDL-cholesterol. For example, if your LDL-cholesterol level is 140 mg/dl and your HDL-cholesterol level is 35 mg/dl, your cholesterol ratio is 140/35 or 4. However, HDL-, LDL-, and total cholesterol levels are independent predictors of your risk for coronary heart disease. Because combining these values into a ratio can conceal information useful to you and your physician, it is more important to know each value separately.

Along with your total blood cholesterol level, your LDL and HDL levels provide more information on your risk of developing coronary heart disease. A high LDL-cholesterol level or a low HDL-cholesterol level puts you at increased risk. LDL- and HDL-cholesterol levels more accurately predict your risk for coronary heart disease than a total cholesterol level alone.

If your doctor measured your LDL-cholesterol level, use the chart below to see how your LDL-cholesterol level measures up.

Desirable	Borderline-High Risk	High Risk
Less than 130 mg/dl	130 to 159 mg/dl	160 mg/dl and above

If your LDL-cholesterol level is in the "desirable" category, you are at an acceptable level of risk. If your LDL level is in the "borderline-high risk" category, you could benefit from lowering your blood cholesterol level by making some dietary changes. If your LDL level is in the "borderline-high risk" category, and you have coronary heart disease or two risk factors for coronary heart disease, you should begin diet treatment under your physician's supervision, as should a person in the "high risk" category. In general, this means you will be paying closer attention to your cholesterol level and making more dietary changes than a person at lower risk.

HDL-cholesterol will also be measured if your total blood cholesterol puts you in a high risk category. The lower your HDL-cholesterol level, the greater your risk for coronary heart disease. Any HDL-cholesterol level lower than 35 mg/dl is considered too low. Quitting smoking, losing weight, and becoming physically active may help raise your HDL-cholesterol level. Although it is not known for certain that raising HDL levels in this way will reduce the risk of coronary heart disease, these measures are likely to be good for your heart in any case.

How to Lower Your High Blood Cholesterol

The primary treatment for high blood cholesterol is a diet that is low in saturated fat and low in cholesterol. This new way of eating is also nutritious, with all the protein, carbohydrate, fat, vitamins, and minerals your body needs. To lower your blood cholesterol, you will:

- Eat less high-fat food (especially those high in saturated fat);
- Replace part of the saturated fat in your diet with unsaturated fat;
- Eat less high-cholesterol food;
- Choose foods high in complex carbohydrates (starch and fiber); and
- Reduce your weight, if you are overweight.

Saturated fats raise your cholesterol level more than anything else in your diet. Dietary cholesterol also raises blood cholesterol levels. Instead of eating foods rich in saturated fat and cholesterol, try more breads, cereals, and other foods high in complex carbohydrates as well as more fruits and vegetables. Using unsaturated fats in place of saturated fats can also help lower your blood cholesterol.

Fortunately, these dietary changes work together. For example, eating less saturated fat may also help you decrease the amount of cholesterol you eat and may help you lose weight. This is because foods high in saturated fat are often high in cholesterol as well and are high in calories. In fact, all fats have more than twice as many calories as either carbohydrate or protein. And, by losing weight if you are overweight, you can help lower your LDL-cholesterol level and increase your HDL-cholesterol level.

Saturated fats are found primarily in animal products, particularly fatty meats and many dairy products. Coconut oil, palm kernel oil, and palm oil are also very saturated. Some of the unsaturated fats in vegetable oils are also made more saturated by a process called hydrogenation. Commercially prepared and processed foods made with these vegetable oils or with saturated fats like butter and lard can also be high in saturated fat.

There are two kinds of unsaturated fat: polyunsaturated and monounsaturated. You should substitute both of these for saturated fat in your diet. Polyunsaturated fats are found primarily in plant products-including safflower, sunflower, corn, soybean, and cottonseed oils; nuts, and seeds-and in fatty fish. Major vegetable oil sources of monounsaturated fats are primarily olive oil and canola oil.

Cholesterol is found only in foods of animal origin, both high-fat foods (like hot dogs and cheddar cheese) and low-fat foods (like liver and other organ meats). And the amount of cholesterol in these foods varies. A daily intake of less than 300 mg is recommended. A 3-ounce piece of meat, fish, or poultry has 60-90 mg of cholesterol; one egg yolk contains about 270 mg; and a 3-ounce serving of liver has about 390 mg of cholesterol.

Again, to reduce your blood cholesterol level, your diet should be low in fat, particularly saturated fat, and low in cholesterol. Use the following guidelines as you plan your new diet.

1. To cut back on saturated fats:
- Choose poultry, fish, and lean cuts of meat more often; remove the skin from chicken and trim the fat from meat.

- Drink skim milk or 1% milk
And eat cheeses with no more than 2-6 grams of fat per ounce (like low-fat cottage or low-fat farmer cheese) instead of processed, natural, and hard cheeses (like American, brie, and cheddar).

- Use tub margarines or liquid vegetable oils that are high in unsaturated fat (like safflower, corn, and olive oil) instead of butter, lard, and hydrogenated vegetable shortening that are high in saturated fat. Choose products that list more unsaturated fat than saturated fat on the label.

- Cut down on commercially prepared and processed foods made with saturated fats or oils. Read labels to choose those low in saturated fats.

2. To cut back on dietary cholesterol:

- Eat less organ meat such as liver, brain, and kidney.
- Eat fewer egg yolks; try substituting two egg whites for each whole egg in recipes.

3. To increase complex carbohydrates (starch and fiber):
- Eat more whole grain breads and cereals, pasta, rice, and dried peas and beans.

- Eat vegetables and fruits more often.

4. To lose weight:

- Eat fewer daily calories (cutting back on fat in your diet will really help).

- Burn extra calories by exercising regularly.

Remember, by closely following your diet and monitoring your progress with regular checkups, you can lower your blood cholesterol level and greatly reduce your risk of developing coronary heart disease.

Generally, both your total and LDL-cholesterol levels will begin to drop 2-3 weeks after you begin your cholesterol-lowering diet. Over time, you may reduce your cholesterol levels by 30-55 mg/dl or even more. The more you reduce your level, the more you will reduce your risk of developing coronary heart disease.

How much you reduce your blood cholesterol levels depends on how much fat, specifically saturated fat, and how much cholesterol you were eating before starting your cholesterol-lowering diet; how well you follow your new diet; and how responsive you body is to the diet. Also, the higher your blood cholesterol level is to begin with, the greater or more dramatic reduction you can expect with your new diet.

Your new cholesterol-lowering diet should be continued for life. While eating some foods high in saturated fat and cholesterol for 1 day or at one meal will not raise blood cholesterol levels, resuming old eating patterns will. Surprisingly, after a while your new way of eating won't seem like a "diet" at all, but simply like your regular routine - full of appealing and appetizing foods.

Before starting your cholesterol-lowering diet, your physician will determine your blood cholesterol goal, specifically the LDL-cholesterol level, that is right for you. This goal will vary depending on whether you have coronary heart disease or any of the other risk factors for coronary heart disease. Even though achieving your LDL-cholesterol goal is more important that the total cholesterol goal, your physician can check your progress by measuring your total cholesterol level because it is a good deal simpler and because you do not have to fast before its measurement. Remember, a total cholesterol level below 200 mg/dl and an LDL-cholesterol below 130 mg/dl are desirable.

To get your blood cholesterol measured, see your doctor or local clinic. They will take a blood sample and send it to a laboratory. There may be differences in your blood cholesterol level from day to day. Cholesterol measurements may also differ somewhat from one laboratory to the next. Your doctor will consider these factors when you return to check your progress. It is important that you have your cholesterol level measured at the same place each time.

Your physician will probably want to measure your cholesterol level after you have been on the diet for 4-6 weeks and again after 3 months. If the total cholesterol goal is met after 3 months, measuring your LDL-cholesterol level will confirm that the LDL-cholesterol goal has been met. If your response to the diet has been satisfactory (both total cholesterol and LDL-cholesterol goals have been met), you will enter a phase of long-term monitoring. Long-term monitoring may involve remeasuring total cholesterol twice a year and LDL-cholesterol once a year.

If you have not met your blood cholesterol goal in 3 months, your doctor may further restrict the saturated fat and cholesterol in your diet and enlist the help of a dietitian. Then, after 4-6 weeks more and again after 3 months, your doctor may measure your cholesterol level. If you have attained your goal, long-term monitoring can begin. If not, your doctor may decide you need medication along with your dietary changes.

Since total cholesterol levels do not change much after a meal, total cholesterol can be measured at any time of day, whether or not you have just eaten. Therefore, you do not need to fast. However, you should not eat or drink anything except water or black coffee for at least 12 hours before having your lipoprotein levels determined (LDL, HDL, triglycerides). Therefore, it may be convenient to eat your last meal at about 9 p.m. and have your test the next day before breakfast.

While dietary change is the first and most important action you will be taking to lower your blood cholesterol level, your doctor may suggest other steps you can take. These will depend on how well the diet lowers your blood cholesterol level and whether or not you have any other risk factors for coronary heart disease.

In most cases, a blood cholesterol-lowering diet is the only step necessary to lower blood cholesterol levels. However, if your LDL-cholesterol level is still too high after you've been on your diet for 6 months, your doctor may decide to include medication as part of your treatment. In addition, if your cholesterol level is unusually high or if you have other major risk factors for coronary heart disease, your doctor may prescribe medications to lower blood cholesterol even sooner.

If your doctor does prescribe medications, you must continue your cholesterol-lowering diet since the combination may allow you to take less medication to lower your levels. And, because diet is still the safest treatment, you should always try to lower your levels with diet alone before adding medication.

There are several medications your physician can prescribe to help you lower your blood cholesterol levels. The report issued by the National Cholesterol Education Program cited the bile acid sequestrants - cholestyramine and colestipol - and nicotinic acids as the drugs of first choice. The report underscored the effectiveness and the long-term safety of these drugs as demonstrated in research studies. The report also cited a new class of drug - HMG CoA reductase - which has demonstrated considerable effectiveness in lowering cholesterol levels. One drug in this class - lovastatin - has been approved for use by the Food and Drug Administration. Because of its newness, long-term safety data has not yet been established. Other drugs cited in the report which were not considered as efficacious in lowering LDL-cholesterol as those mentioned above include gemfibrozil and probucol. All cholesterol-lowering medication should be taken only with the advice of and under supervision of your physician.

The key changes you need to make are the ones discussed above. To review:

- Follow a diet that is low in saturated fat and cholesterol. This is the most important step you will take to help reduce your high blood cholesterol level.

- Maintain a desirable weight. If you need to lose weight, your new diet will help since it is likely to be lower in calories than your current diet.
- Finally, exercise to help you lose weight and improve your overall physical fitness. Exercise may also help you raise your HDL level.

Unless your doctor prescribes a cholesterol-lowering medication, these are the only steps you will need to take to lower your blood cholesterol level.

Fortunately, you can do something about all three of the major risk factors for coronary heart disease - high blood cholesterol, cigarette smoking, and high blood pressure. Thus, in addition to lowering your blood cholesterol level, it is a good idea to quit smoking and control your blood pressure. Maintaining your desirable weight will also help you lower your risk for coronary heart disease. And all of these steps will help you to feel better.

Need more help? Want to know more? There are many places you can go to get information about your new diet, your diagnosis, and the latest findings about treatment and medications for high blood cholesterol.

If you want some help following your recommended diet, talk to a registered dietitian or qualified nutritionist. They can explain the diet to you in greater detail and show you ways to follow it. They can give you advice on shopping and preparing foods, eating away from home, and changing your eating habits to help you stay on your new diet. They will also help you set goals for dietary change so that you can successfully lower your high blood cholesterol levels without drastically changing your eating pattern and overall lifestyle all at one time. The

Division of Practice of the American Dietetic Association [(312) 899-0040] can help you find a registered dietitian in your area. State and local branches of the American Dietetic Association, your local hospital, or your doctor can recommend a dietitian for you.

There are also other resources. The nurse in your doctor's office can answer questions you may have about your high blood cholesterol or your new diet. If your blood cholesterol level is not lowered within a reasonable amount of time, your doctor may refer you to a physician who is a lipid specialist. Lipid specialists are experts in the management of high blood cholesterol and other lipid disorders. If you have questions about drug therapy or the medication your doctor is prescribing, ask your doctor. Finally, pharmacists are also aware of the best ways to take medication, of ways to minimize side effects, and of the latest research about specific drugs.

If you would like more information to help you start your new approach to healthy eating, contact the National Cholesterol Education Program (NCEP) of the National Heart, Lung, and Blood Institute. Another NCEP pamphlet that can help you, Eating to Lower Your High Blood Cholesterol, provides more specific information on how to lower your blood cholesterol levels through diet. NCEP also has developed a resource list of agencies and organizations that can answer your questions. These and other materials can be requested by writing to the National Cholesterol Education Program, National Heart, Lung, and Blood Institute, C-200, Bethesda, MD 20892.

GLOSSARY

1. **Atherosclerosis** - A type of "hardening of the arteries" in which cholesterol, fat, and other blood components build up in the walls of arteries. As atherosclerosis progresses, the arteries to the heart may narrow so that oxygen-rich blood and nutrients have difficulty reaching the heart.

2. **Bile acid sequestrants** - One type of cholesterol-lowering medication, including cholestyramine and colestipol. The sequestrants bind with cholesterol-containing bile acids in the intestine and remove them in bowel movements.

3. **Carbohydrate** - One of the three nutrients that supply calories (energy) to the body. Carbohydrate provides 4 calories per gram - the same number of calories as pure protein and less than half the calories of fat. Carbohydrate is essential for normal body function. There are two basic kinds of carbohydrate - simple carbohydrate (or sugars) and complex carbohydrate (starches and fiber). In nature, both the simple sugars and the complex starches come packaged in foods like oranges, apples, corn, wheat, and milk. Refined or processed carbohydrates are found in cookies, cakes, and pies.

   - **Complex carbohydrate** - Starch and fiber. Complex carbohydrate comes from plants. When complex carbohydrate is substituted for saturated fat, the saturated fat reduction lowers blood cholesterol. Foods high in starch include breads, cereals, pasta, rice, dried beans and peas, corn, and lima beans.

   - **Fiber** - A nondigestible type of complex carbohydrate. High-fiber foods are usually low in calories. Foods high in fiber include whole grain breads and cereals, whole fruits, and dried beans. The type of fiber found in foods such as oat and barley bran, some fruits like apples and oranges, and some dried beans may help reduce blood cholesterol.

4. **Cholesterol** - A soft, waxy substance. It is made in sufficient quantity by the body for normal body function, including the manufacture of hormones, bile acid, and vitamin D. It is present in all parts of the body, including the nervous system, muscle, skin, liver, intestines, heart, etc.

- **Blood cholesterol** - Cholesterol that is manufactured in the liver and absorbed from the food you eat and is carried in the blood for use by all parts of the body. A high level of blood cholesterol leads to atherosclerosis and coronary heart disease.

- **Dietary cholesterol** - cholesterol that is in the food you eat. It is present only in foods of animal origin, not in foods of plant origin. Dietary cholesterol, like dietary saturated fat, tends to raise blood cholesterol, which increases the risk for heart disease.

5. **Coronary heart disease** - Heart ailment caused by narrowing of the coronary arteries (arteries that supply oxygen and nutrients directly to the heart muscle). Coronary heart disease is caused by atherosclerosis, which decreases the blood supply to the heart muscle. The inadequate supply of oxygen-rich blood and nutrients damages the heart muscle and can lead to chest pain, heart attack, and death.

6. **Fat** - One of the three nutrients that supply calories to the body. Fat provides 9 calories per gram, more than twice the number

provided by carbohydrate or protein. In addition to providing calories, fat helps in the absorption of certain vitamins. Small amounts of fat are necessary for normal body function.

- **Total fat** - The sum of the saturated, monounsaturated, and polyunsaturated fats present in food. A mixture of all three in varying amounts is found in most foods.

- **Saturated fat** - A type of fat found in greatest amounts in foods from animals such as meat, poultry, and whole-milk dairy products like cream, milk, ice cream, and cheese,. Other examples of saturated fat include butter, the marbling and fat along the edges of meat and lard, and the saturated fat content is high in some vegetable oils like coconut, palm kernel, and palm oils. Saturated fat raises blood cholesterol more than anything else in the diet.

- **Unsaturated fat** - A type of fat that is usually liquid at refrigerator temperature. Monounsaturated fat and polyunsaturated fat are two kinds of unsaturated fat.

- **Monounsaturated fat** - A slightly unsaturated fat that is found in greatest amounts in foods from plants, including olive and canola (rapeseed) oil. When substituted for saturated fat, Monounsaturated fat helps reduce blood cholesterol.

- **Polyunsaturated fat** - A highly unsaturated fat that is found in greatest amounts in foods from plants, including safflower, sunflower, corn and soybean oil. When substituted for saturated fat, polyunsaturated fat helps reduce blood cholesterol.

7. **Gram (g)** - A unit of weight. There are about 28 g in 1 ounce. Dietary fat, protein, and carbohydrate are measured in grams.

8. **Hydrogenation** - A chemical process that changes liquid vegetable oils (unsaturated fat) into a more solid saturated fat. This process improves the shelf life of the product but also increases the saturated fat content. Many commercial food products contain hydrogenated vegetable oil. Selection should be made based on information found on the label.

9. **Lipids** - Fatty substances, including cholesterol and triglycerides, that are present in blood and body tissues.

10. **Lipoproteins** - Protein-coated packages that carry fat and cholesterol through the blood. Lipoproteins are classified according to their density.

- **High density lipoproteins (HDL)** - Lipoproteins that contain a small amount of cholesterol and carry cholesterol away from body cells and tissues to the liver for excretion from the body. Low levels of HDL are associated with an increased risk of coronary heart disease. Therefore, the higher the HDL level, the better.

- **Low density lipoproteins (LDL)** - Lipoproteins that contain the largest amount of cholesterol in the blood. LDL is responsible for depositing cholesterol in the artery walls. High levels of LDL are associated with an increased risk or coronary heart disease and are therefore referred to as "bad cholesterol".

11. **Milligram (mg)** - A unit of weight equal to one thousandth of a gram. There are about 28,350 mg in 1 ounce. Dietary cholesterol is measured in milligrams.

12. Milligrams/deciliter (mg/dl) - A way of expressing concentration: in blood cholesterol measurements, the weight of cholesterol (in milligrams) in a deciliter of blood. A deciliter is about one-tenth of a quart.

13. Niacin - A B vitamin essential for energy production in cells. The recommended daily allowance is about 14 mg for adult females and about 18 mg for adult males. When used in massive quantities under a physician's guidance, niacin in considered a cholesterol-lowering medication.

14. Protein - One of the three nutrients that supply calories to the body. Protein provides 4 calories per gram, which is less than half the calories of fat. Protein is an essential nutrient that becomes a component of many parts of the body, including muscle, bone, skin, and blood.

15. Risk factor - A habit, trait, or condition in a person that is associated with an increased chance of developing a disease.

16. Triglycerides - Lipids (fat-like substances) carried through the bloodstream to the tissues. The bulk of the body's fat tissue is in the form of triglycerides, stored for later use as energy. We get triglycerides primarily from the fat in our diet.

17. Vascular disease - An ailment of the blood vessels often caused by atherosclerosis. Vascular disease may occur in the arteries to the brain and the major leg arteries.

Chapter 7
Eating Out

Trends in Eating Out

Americans are on the move. Busy lifestyles and tight work and travel schedules make eating out routine for many of us. According to recent surveys:

- Americans, excluding those who live in institutions, eat more than one of every five meals at away-from-home eating establishments.

- Fast-food places serve 4 out of 10 meals eaten at away-from-home eating establishments.

- Four out of 10 consumers say they have changed their eating habits to reflect nutritional concerns.

- Adults eat roughly 30 percent of their calories away from home.

- Americans spend more than 40 cents of every food dollar on food eaten away from home.

What Guidelines Should You Follow When Eating Out or At Home?

The dietary guidelines for Americans are seven basic principles for developing and maintiaining a healthier diet. The Guidelines represent the best thinking in the field of nutrition information and education programs for healthy Americans. They were developed by the U.S. Department of Agriculture and the U.S. Department of Health and Humans Services.

The Dietary Guidelines emphasize balance, variety, and moderation in the overall diet. The seven Guidelines are:

- Eat a variety of foods
- Maintain desirable weight (Body fat content)
- Avoid too much fat, saturated fat, and cholesterol
- Eat foods with adequate starch and fiber
- Avoid too much sugar
- Avoid too much sodium
- If you drink alcoholic beverages, do so in moderation

How does eating out affect your overall diet? That depends on where you eat, what, and how much you order, and what extras you add to the foods you order - dressings, spreads, condiments, and so forth. Of course, how often you eat out is important, too.

Where you eat out greatly affects the food choices available to you. It is a lot easier to follow Guidelines-style eating at some restaurants than at other. For example, a greater selection of menu items gives you the opportunity to choose for variety. And if foods are prepared to order, you can have more control over the calories, fat, sugars, and sodium in your meal. Here's how eating places compare:

Full service restaurants usually provide the greatest variety and flexibility in types of foods and preparation methods. Items are often prepared to order, so you can ask that foods be prepared differently than the menu specifies.

One drawback of having foods prepared to order is the time it takes - what and how much do you eat while waiting for your order?

For lunch in Kansas City, I choose The Soup Exchange because they offer good tasting, fat-free menu items.

For dinner (supper to some) I might choose Bob Gaines Colony Steak House and Lobster Pot. I simply call ahead and tell them that I'm bringing my own butter and salad dressing. That is never a problem. When I arrive and order, I simply give my server a packet of Butter Buds® flavor granules so it can be served with my lobster.

When my salad arrives, I whip out my small bottle of fat-free salad dressing and enjoy. Later, my boiled Main lobster arrives with its bubbling hot "butter" for my baked potato and to dip my lobster in. I am apparently eating what everyone else is eating, however, my meal is essentially fat free!

If I crave bar-b-que in Kansas City, I choose the Smokestack Restaurant in Martin City. They grill everthing over an open fire. I usually choose fire-grilled skinless boneless breast of chicken or fish, vegetable kebob also grilled, ranch beans (similar to recipe on page 261), and a tossed green salad with my own fat-free salad dressing. I simply ask that nothing is to basted in butter or grease and I go real light on the wonderful beans. I am never deprived nor do I stick out of the crowd. (I have my wife hide the dressing in her purse).

Cafeterias, smorgasbords, and restaurant buffets also provide a wide variety of food selections. Since foods are prepared in advance, there's no wait, but you are not able to order foods the way you want them. You do, however, have some control over portion size and the amounts of sauces, gravies, and dressings served with foods. Watch out for "all-you-can-eat" offers, though. You may be tempted to eat too much just to get your money's worth! Also, many cafeterias have fallen in love with butter flavored oil which sometimes shows up in all of their vegetable dishes. Check it out! If it looks like green beans are swimming in grease then they probably are.

Pizza parlors offer variety in toppings and crust types but an otherwise limited menu. Toppings vary in calories, fat, and sodium content. Some parlors feature salad bars. In Kansas City, Gino Shiraldi's Pizza Company will always fix me a pizza with extra mushrooms, tomatoes, jalapenos, and some beef topping. I ask them to hold the cheese and oil and I end up with a super pizza. The beef topping at most pizza parlors contains TVP® and is much lower in fat than pepperoni or Italian sausage.

Convenience store "mini-meals" and vending machines are a growing source of food eaten away from home. Offerings include chili, hotdogs and Polish sausages, nachos with cheese sauce, prepackaged hamburgers and sandwiches, single-serving foods, candy, and snack foods. Fat, calories, sugars, and sodium are high in many of these items, expecially in processed, prepackaged, and canned foods. Some refrigerated vending machines offer alternatives - yogurt, fruit, and fruit juices, for example.

Other people's homes can provide a real challenge to eating in the Guidelines style. How much control you have (or are willing to take) may depend on several factors, including the risk of offending your host or hostess! Buffet arrangements and informal parties permit you to be selective in what and how much you choose. However, there is often a tempting array of food and drinks that are high in fat, sugars, sodium, or alcohol. Family-style dinners may make it more difficult to avoid certain food selection, but you can still control serving sizes. Of course, formal sit-down dinners, where you're served a prepared plate of food, provide you with the least control.

When people invite me to their homes to eat they understand that I have an on-going battle with fat, so they always make provisions, usually in the form of breast of chicken, shrimp, or scallops.

I suggest that when you are invited for dinner, be your own advocate and inform the person asking that you are, of necessity, on a very low fat diet and inquire if this would cause embarassment or undue problems. If not, then accept and enjoy the chicken.

Sub shops offer a varied selection of subs and sandwiches but usually little else. Items are prepared to order so the amount of high-calorie, high-fat spreads can be limited. Sometimes smaller servings are available. Many offer a variety of breads.

Just make sure to stick to breast of turkey, breast of chicken, or lean beef. Skip the bologna, salami, and other, fat meats.

Fast food restaurants offer an expanding but still rather limited menu. Many items are deep-fat fried, including chicken and fish items, french fries, onion rings, and fruit pies. However, smaller servings are available for some sandwiches and side orders, and you can request that foods be prepared without sauces or other condiments. Salads, baked potatoes, and whole-grain rolls are now available at some fast-food restaurants, and lowfat milk and fruit juices are joining soft drinks and shakes as beverage options.

Ask for a copy of the nutrition information sheet that most fast-food restaurants companies now offer. You'll be plesantly surprised to find many with very low fat items. Beware of mexican food because they still insist on adding fat to refried beans, Spanish rice and tortillas.

Chapter 8
Time for Tea

Since we all snack, I make a motion that we reinstitute the traditional English tea time. Let's call it a special calm time.

If I were a young housewife, I would definitely set aside time each afternoon from 2:00 to 2:30 p.m. for tea (or coffee) and a special tidbit, purposefully prepared for my special time. I would invite child, mate, neighbor, or friend to attend and participate. I would buy a variety pack of teas and/or different coffees and I would choose from the following list of spreads, breads, scones, and cakes.

Breads, Cakes & Spreads

1. Salt Rising Pumpkin Bread, page 257
1. Cream Cheese, page 322
2. Irish Soda Bread, page 269
2. Apple Butter
3. Scones, page 273
3. Orange Marmalade
4. Salt Rising Tea Bread, page 255
4. Tuna Spread, page 100
5. Baked Custard Crusts, page 289
5. Smoked Turkey Spread, page 101
6. Cake, page 290 through page 306

My rules for tea time would be as follows:

Rule #1 - You must be prompt. Tardiness will not be tolerated. Tea time will bring consistency into my life, something that I can count on.

Rule #2 - You must engage in intelligent conversation, or if alone, indulge in thoughtful reading or just relax and let your mind become calm.

Rule #3 - No television of any sort.

Rule #4 - Turn the radio on to calm background music whether alone or with guests.

Rule #5 - Teach pre-schoolers to participate and enjoy tea time if awake.

Rule #6 - Only no fat foods allowed.

Rule #7 - You must relax and enjoy your own great food.

This kind of break would also be beneficial in the corporate or small business setting.

Chapter 9

Soybeans and Soy Products - A Rich Source of Protein

Over 4,000 years ago, the Chinese discovered the value of the soybean as a readily available source of edible protein. Yet in the United States, the soybean's enormous potential as a nutritional resource remained virtually untapped until the 1920s, when U.S. farmers first began growing soybean crops in commercial quantities. Today more soybeans are grown in the United States than anywhere else in the world. In 1990, about 440,000 U.S. soybean farmers harvested 1.9 billion bushels of soybeans.

In a world faced with exponential population growth and rapidly dwindling resources, the soybean may provide a much-needed dietary miracle. It converts nutrients from the soil into quality edible protein with incredible efficiency, and it is the single largest nutritive source of both protein and oil in the world. Food technologists have extracted from the soybean an economical and highly nutritious food resource: soy protein.

The comparative cost of soy protein is significantly lower than other protein sources. For example, the cost of protein in ground beef is more than twenty times the cost of soy protein.

Furthermore, soy protein is acknowledged to be the highest quality form of vegetable protein and is one of the most abundant. The world produces more than 60 million metric tons of soybeans each year. The amount of soy protein produced per acre of land is a good indication of the soybean's value as a highly efficient source of edible protein.

For example, beef cattle grazing on one acre of land can produce 58 pounds of edible protein, enough to sustain a person for 77 days. The same acre planted in wheat can yield 180 pounds of protein, enough to sustain a person for 877 days. Yet one acre of soybeans can furnish 584 pounds of edible protein, enough to sustain an individual for 2,224 days.

Today thousands of soy protein products are on the supermarket shelves; they range from baby foods and formula to delicious entrees like cholesterol-free all vegetable Midland Harvest® Brand Burgers.

Midland Harvest Burgers® are becoming more and more available in supermarkets. If you can't find them in your supermarket, you can still order them by telephoning Harvest Direct, Inc. at 1-800-8-FLAVOR. This company also carries a full line of TVP® varieties.

TVP® is made by extruding or texturizing defatted soy flour. TVP® is practically fat free and approaches the texture and chewy quality of meat. I have been involved in some serious debates over whether my Chile Con Carne and Spaghetti "meat" sauce were really fat free and truly meatless; they were, due entirely to the use of TVP®.

Here is a list of some varieties available:
(a) Ground Beef
(b) Strip Beef Style
(c) Chunk Beef Style
(d) Ground Poultry Style
(e) Chunk Poultry Style
(f) Flavored Ground Beef Style
(g) Flavored Chunk Beef Style
(h) Bacon Style Bits.

Midland Harvest Burger® and TVP® are registered trademarks of Archer Daniels Midland Company and are used with permission.

" Take thou also unto thee wheat, and barley, and beans, and lentiles, and millet and fitches, and put them in one vessel and make bread there of......"

Ezekiel 4:9

Chapter 10

Venison*

In the year 1992, dramatic new evidence indicates that humans had crossed the Bering straits and migrated at least as far south as Ft. Bliss (El Paso) Texas by the year 28,000 B.C. and perhaps as early as 38,000 B.C. Those folks as well as all other humans of that period had adapted to a diet rich in vegetables, fruits, grains, grass seeds, and wild game. This was a diet very low in fat.

Most wild game is very lean due to the inability of the muscle meat to become marbled. As with turkey and chicken, wild game will become fat around the muscle, but not inside the muscle. Hence, when the exterior fat is removed, you've removed almost all of the fat.

For those who must have red meat in their diet, I strongly suggest you consider and include some New Zealand farm raised venison. Venison will allow you to return to one of the meat staples of your ancestors, a staple you were designed to operate on, a staple that will help you burn brightly before you flicker.

Venison can be obtained by calling Game Sales International, Inc. at 1 (303) 667-4090.

Once the fare of royalty, venison has recently gained new visibility and popularity among a growing number of chefs in America. These chefs are aiming to please discriminating diners on the lookout for healthy, flavorful alternatives to cholesterol-laden meats and high-calorie entrees.

Venison has been eaten for centuries, yet its nutritional benefits are a perfect match for an increasingly health-conscious modern society.

* Some information provided by The New Zealand Farm Raised Venison Council, Oakland, California.

71

This distinctive meat is higher in protein and lower in fat and cholesterol than lean beef, white or dark turkey meat, skinned chicken breasts, and even many seafoods.

Venison is often assumed to be a heavy, gamey tasting meat obtained from deer captured in the wild. Actually, the majority of all venison served in restaurants around the world today comes from grass-fed deer raised on farms in New Zealand. The meat is delightfully mild, but flavorful, and extremely tender when prepared properly.

A NOBLE HISTORY

Today's farm raised venison is a modern commodity that has evolved from an age-old tradition. Deer have been hunted by man since prehistoric times and were an important source not only for food, but for tools and weapons fashioned from the antlers and bones of the deer.

European nobles depended on deer herds as a source of nourishment for their troops, but eventually cattle became more important for this purpose because they provided the high fat content essential to soldiers who needed energy to stay warm during the winters.

For this same reason, beef became a food of peasants while the leaner venison became a "royal food" for the gentry, who lived in warm, protected homes.

The influence of the early aristocratic connoisseurs of venison is still evident today in the type of venison dishes most commonly served by the world's finest restaurants. Royal palates preferred hearty, rich dishes. Lengthy marinating and heavy sauces were long considered necessary to increase the tenderness of the meat and cover up the "wild game" flavor and any inconsistencies created by the animal's age, composition and diet, however this is not necessary with farm raised venison.

DEER INTRODUCED TO NEW ZEALAND

Deer were not found in New Zealand until the 19th century when the islands became a British colony. In the late 1800s and early 1900s, deer were brought to New Zealand from English parks and Scottish highlands to provide game for the English sportsmen who had settled there. No deer herds were native to New Zealand, but once introduced, the animals thrived under the ideal conditions -- mild climate, plentiful food and no natural predators.

Eventually, the rapidly multiplying herds became a problem. Hunters could not kill the deer quickly enough to stave off the problems they were creating in the forest and for farmers. These wild deer were causing a serious erosion problem and depleting the feed supplies on the lower hills, creating a food shortage for local livestock.

From the 1930s until the beginning of World War II, the government enlisted professional hunters to shoot the deer to stabilize the population and control the massive growth. The problem abated until the hunting was stopped during the war. Once again, the surplus deer became a problem.

In the 1960s, a few entrepreneurs recognized an opportunity to ship the deer to Europe where venison was traditionally a favored dish. Deer hunting eventually became so lucrative and sophisticated that helicopters were used as a foolproof method of recovering the animals.

Export tonnages surged to a peak of nearly 10,000,000 lbs. in 1972. Ironically, once the European market for New Zealand venison was highly developed, supply began to be a problem. So many deer had been killed that the wild herds were diminished to a point where helicopter hunting could not longer support the rapidly increasing number of operators.

Reluctant to turn their backs on a lucrative business opportunity, exporters turned to deer farming as a way to ensure future supplies of venison to newly developed markets. Helicopter operators switched from shooting deer to capturing them as foundation breeding stock for deer farms.

MODERN-DAY DEER FARMING IN NEW ZEALAND

The first license for a deer farm was issued in March, 1970. Today, there are more than a million and a half deer on more than 5,000 deer farms throughout New Zealand.

Initially, New Zealand exported its product mainly to West Germany and European countries. But in the past 10 years, there has been a demand for venison in the United States. From 1976 to 1984, imports of New Zealand venison increased from 175,000 pounds to 600,000 pounds, with an estimated 1.5 million pounds of exports of New Zealand venison, importing 1.2 million pounds, up 43% from 1989.

The deer are slaughtered in New Zealand, butchered and conveniently packaged in an array of meat cuts to ship worldwide. More than 60 percent of the product today is shipped chill-packed for freshness. In the United States, venison is sold primarily to restaurants, but also increasingly to a growing number of specialty gourmet shops and meat stores in major cities.

U.S. chefs are beginning to recognize that venison offers substantial health benefits to Americans who love red meat, but who are becoming more concerned about trimming high fat and cholesterol diets. Surprisingly, venison is lower in fat, cholesterol and calories than beef, skinned chicken breast, light or dark turkey meat and baked salmon. In fact, venison offers 50 percent more protein than lean beef, with only half the calories.

Chefs at trendy, upscale American restaurants are experimenting with new ways of preparing venison, sans the heavy, rich, caloric sauces of the past. Some of the new dishes now available are: venison salads, grilled venison, venison kebabs, cajun-style venison, etc.

Evolving from a food of kings to a food of the upscale and nutrition-conscious, venison promises to become a popular item in the American diet.

Cuts Available:

1. Hind leg cuts can be purchased bone-in or boneless. Boneless leg cuts include topside, thick flank, rump and silverside. Shoulder cuts are available mainly in boneless form and can be purchased as shepherd steaks or diced from many suppliers.

2. Both shoulders and legs are good for steaks, schnitzels, kebabs, roasts, stirfries, grills, sautes, meatballs, sausages and pies.

3. The saddle is traditionally considered the premier quality venison cut, offering the highest quality and requiring little trimming. Saddle is good for roasts, steaks or fillets.

Preparation:

1. Keep raw meat refrigerated on a covered plate. Don't use plastic -- the meat should not sweat.

2. Carefully remove any sinew or skin before pan "frying" or grilling. (Many cuts can be purchased fully desinewed.) Boneless cuts need to be separated into individual pieces by following the seam of each muscle and removing the silverskin. It is crucial to remove the muscle coating skin for tender, quality steaks.

3. Always slice meat across the grain, not with it.

4. Allow up to 6-8 ounces of meat per main course serving and about 3-4 ounces for smaller entree portions and small plates.

5. Cook venison quickly, on high heat.

6. Always serve venison rare or medium rare - because it is a lean meat. Medium or well-done venison can be tough and dry, unless cooked tender as in a stew.

7. Cook steaks, medallions and sautes at the last minute when everything else is ready.

8. Never attempt to reheat venison except as an addition to the stew pot.

9. A marinade involves three elements -- acid, seasonings and oil. The acid assists in tenderizing the meat, herbs, spices and

seasonings act to impart complementary flavors and oil will allow the transfer of flavors through the meat. When marinating venison skip the oil and:

Marinate small cuts only briefly to complement flavor.

Marinate large cuts no longer than four hours.

Try wine, vinegar, lemon juice, beer or buttermilk as a marinade for juicy venison steaks.

Tart fruits, such as kiwi fruit, pineapple and raspberry, make excellent marinades for venison.

Serving Ideas:

1. Venison is excellent as steaks, roasts, charcoaled or in kebabs, gyros, ragouts, salads and sandwiches.

2. Serve New Zealand venison kebabs, patties or stir fires with black rice, wild rice or baked vegetables such as kumeras or potatoes.

3. Make mountain man sandwiches with large loaves of french bread: fill with grilled, or roast venison, steaks or patties, plum sauce or chutney, sour cream, sprouts and sliced tomato.

4. Serve barbecued venison with beer, champagne or a chilled Gerwerztraminer.

5. Use tart fruits as accompaniments in sauces for venison, or as light marinades to accent flavor.

6. When venison dishes are richly sauced, serve noodles or bland potatoes as accompaniment.

7. Accompany New Zealand venison dishes with a range of sweet to dry wines to suit your cooking style -- often white wines enhance venison dishes.

8. Venison can be grilled over mesquite, stir-fried, wind-dried, roasted and sauteed.

9. Venison is also tasty when served blackened Cajun-style.

10. Use venison to give Southwestern dishes an authentic and flavorful twist.

11. Venison can be a unique pasta filling for tortellini or ravioli.

CHARCOALED MESQUITE VENISON STEAKS

Make sure everything else for your meal is ready and on the table before starting to cook your steaks.

Individual steaks are fine but I like to cook one big thick steak and then slice it in 1/4" slices at the table.

Season your steaks with salt, pepper or your favorite seasoned salt or a salt-free herb seasoning mix then place them over a hot mesquite charcoal fire and cook to a rare or medium rare doneness.

Note: for a real New Mexico treat dust each steak with a generous amount of chili powder or dry enchilada mix before charcoaling. Serve with Spanish rice page 170 and warm tortillas.

SOUTHWESTERN MESQUITE SMOKED VENISON

Generously coat a venison roast with chile powder, some salt and insert a meat thermometer. Place meat on charcoal grill away from the direct heat of the charcoal and cover allowing the smoke to circulate around the roast. Add wet mesquite wood chips periodically to create smoke. When thermometer indicates rare or medium rare, remove and serve immediately. This smoking may take several hours. If impatience sets in move meat closer to hot coals to expedite cooking.

HICKORY CAJUN VENISON STEAKS

Generously powder steaks with your favorite blackening spices and place them over a hot bed of hickory charcoal. Grill until rare or medium rare and serve immediately.

Note: Can be cooked inside on a cast iron griddle or heavy skillet. Just be sure to cook steaks quickly. Serve with a baked potato, sour cream and chives and a hearty warm bread.

VENISON SWISS STEAK

1 1/2   pounds venison round steaks
1/2   cup tomatoes, canned, chopped
1/4   cup onions chopped
1/4   cup beef stock or water
         Vegetable spray
         Season to taste

Pound steaks to tenderize and cut into serving size pieces. In dutch oven or heavy skillet that has been veggie sprayed brown steaks. Add remaining ingredients. Cover and simmer for 1 1/2 hours until tender. Stir often.

PINEAPPLE TERIYAKI VENISON

1   pound venison cut into 1 inch cubes
1/2   cup teriyaki sauce
1   cup pineapple chunks

1/2   cup pineapple juice
1/2   tablespoon cornstarch
       Vegetable spray

In dutch oven or heavy skillet that has been veggie sprayed, brown venison, add teriyaki sauce and pineapple chunks and simmer until meat is done medium rare (5-10 minutes) meanwhile mix pineapple juice and cornstarch together and pour over meat. When thickened, serve over steamed rice.

HUNTER'S STEW (VENISON)

4 or 5 servings

1   pound venison, cut into 1 inch cubes
3 or 4   medium potatoes
1   small to medium onion, chopped
1   can beef broth
3   cups water
2   tablespoons flour
         Vegetable spray

Veggie spray a dutch oven or heavy skillet, add meat and brown. Sprinkle 1 tablespoon flour over meat and bottom of pan. Stir and continue browning until flour turns dark brown but not burnt. Add 1/2 can of beef broth a spoonful at a time as the browning continues. When well browned add water and onions cover and simmer until meat is tender. Add potatoes and continue simmering until potatoes are tender, about 30 minutes.

Meanwhile mix 1 tablespoon flour and 1/2 can beef broth and pour into meat and potatoes. When thickened serve with fresh warm bread.

VENISON SMOTHERED IN ONIONS

1	pound venison steak
2	medium onions, sliced
	Flour
1	can beef broth
1	teaspoon vinegar
1/4	teaspoon thyme
1	small bay leaf
1	teaspoon parsley
1/2	teaspoon garlic
	Water
	Vegetable spray
	Salt and pepper to taste

Over medium/high temperature in a veggie sprayed dutch oven or heavy skillet place onions on one side, and 1 teaspoon flour over the other side and brown. When flour is brown add floured and seasoned steak. Brown meat and turn over. To hasten browning, add a little beef broth, vinegar, thyme, bay leaf, parsley, garlic and enough water to just cover the meat. Reduce temperature to where the meat is just simmering and cook for about 2 hours until meat is tender. Serve, topped with onions, with mashed potatoes, page 169, your veggie choice and warm fresh bread.

VENISON-ONION ROAST
(Courtesy of Judy Hall, Lenexa, Kansas)

1   Two or three pound venison roast
1   Packet onion soup mix
     Vegetable spray

Preheat oven to 350 degrees F. Brown roast in veggie sprayed dutch oven. Sprinkle with soup mix and cover with water. Bake until tender.

Chapter 11

Buffalo

It tastes like the best beef you've ever eaten! Forget gamey, sweet, or other peculiar descriptive words. It simply tastes like a well-aged prime piece of beef and if you spring a cookout featuring "T" bones, rare to medium rare, your guests will wolf them down with thanksgiving gusto. Now if you don't tell them what they are eating, they will undoubtedly enjoy it more and be the better for it. Even when you've gone so far as to let your guests select their steak, they will marvel at the attractiveness of the meat and relish the flavor. The brain isn't always helpful when it comes to something "different" but if you crave red meat and the doctor says "No - no," then you should definitely consider buffalo. Here is why:

70% less fat and 50% less cholesterol.

How is this possible?

The benefits of buffalo meat lie in the basic nature and biological or genetic attributes of buffalo.

Buffalo do not marble!

"Marble", meaning to put fat in the muscle. When you see a lean cut of buffalo, you can believe that it is lean. About 97.2% lean, or just under 1 gram of fat per ounce of roasted lean meat (according to the Human Nutrition Information Service of the USDA). The fat content of lean buffalo meat puts it in the same category with chicken or turkey breast meat. However, buffalo clearly wins the cholesterol battle. Three ounces of roasted buffalo has just 39 mg of cholesterol compared to breast meat chicken at 73 mg, turkey breast at 72 mg and beef at 79 mg. For you "clogged artery" folks, buffalo makes a lot of sense, and it should make sense for those who don't have or want clogged arteries.

Where to Buy
Telephone: Game Sales International, Inc.
Denver, Colorado
1-303-667-4090
Or Contact: American Bison Association
1-303-292-2833
In Kansas City, I buy my buffalo from:
McGonigles Market, 1307 W. 79th Street

Cooking Tips

Buffalo is cooked in much the same way you would cook beef with only a couple of important differences. You can't cook a buffalo steak "well done" because it gets tough and if cooking stews or soups it takes longer for the buffalo to reach the tender stage. Steaks or roasts should be "rare" or "medium rare".

The lack of fat guarantees that your buffalo will cook faster than beef. Since fat is an insulation, and not present in buffalo, the meat cooks quicker. Well marbled beef cooks slower, pound for pound than lean commercial grade beef. Since buffalo lacks marbling the meat has a tendency to be done well before what you are used to. In this regard, it takes some trial and error to effectively master this quick cooking phenomenon.

When broiling buffalo move your rack about a notch farther away from the heat, that way it will be done in about the same amount of time.

If you would normally roast your beef at 325 degrees F, turn the heat down to 275 degrees F for buffalo and plan on the roast being done in about the same amount of time.

When roasting, always use a meat thermometer and remove when "rare" to "medium rare" for best results.

Ground buffalo is also leaner than what you are used to. You should figure about 10% fat or in a 1/4 pounder that means about 11 grams of fat per serving. The thicker the patty the juicer the meat.

A very interesting taste experience evolves with the combining of chicken broth and buffalo. I demonstrate that in the green chile burrito and the smothered minute steaks. I don't think any finer flavored foods are available anywhere, and for them to be healthy and good for you is an amazing extra.

Steaks recommended for grilling include minute steaks, rib eyes, T-bones, and New York strips:

Sear both sides of your steak on hot grill to keep the juices in the steak, then you can lower the heat on the stove or move the meat to a cooler spot on the outdoor grill.

Don't use a fork when turning meat; use tongs instead, that way the juices stay inside your steak.

When cooking a roast, low temperatures and moist heat is recommended. Remember your roast is best either rare or medium rare. The next step after medium rare requires a lot of cooking time to reach the "fork tender" stage.

Don't be apprehensive about preparing buffalo. Use as a direct substitute for fatty beef and have a healthier heart for your effort. Enjoy.

GREEN CHILE BUFFALO BURRITO

1   pound buffalo meat cut into small bite-size pieces
1   can chicken broth
2   anaheim green chile peppers, chopped
1   medium onion, chopped
        Salt and pepper to taste
        Water to process

In sauce pan brown meat. Add chicken broth, 1/2 of the green pepper and 1/2 of the onion. Simmer for hours, adding water as needed, until "fork tender". Cook down the juice until the bottom of pan is just covered and add remaining peppers and onions. Continue to simmer until peppers are tender. Season and serve with warm flour tortillas.

ONION SMOTHERED BUFFALO MINUTE STEAKS
(for 2)

2   minute steaks tenderized, seasoned, and floured
1   large onion, sliced
1   can chicken broth, defatted
        Flour
        Salt and pepper to taste
        Vegetable spray

In large veggie-sprayed skillet on medium-high heat, place onion slices and grill for 2 or 3 minutes, push over to one side and splash on top of onions 3 or 4 tablespoons chicken broth. Place steaks in skillet and brown. After turning once, splash on several tablespoons of broth under steaks, allow to cook off and brown but not burn. Mix 1 tablespoon of flour to remaining broth. Stir until smooth and pour into skillet. Stir as gravy thickens. Remove steaks when just barely done to your satisfaction. Top with onions and gravy and serve.

MESQUITE SMOKED BUFFALO ROAST

Buffalo roast with all visible fat removed
Salt and pepper to taste

On outdoor grill, place roast that has been peppered (but not salted yet) away from mesquite fire. Cover grill and allow to smoke meat for at least an hour. Place roast over fire and allow to brown on all sides and add salt. When you think that the meat is about done, insert meat thermometer. When center of meat is rare to medium rare, remove and serve.

RED CHILE CON CARNE BUFFALO FOR TWO

1   pound buffalo roast, cut into bite-size pieces
1   dry red chile, seeds removed
     Water to process
     Salt to taste

In heavy sauce pan or dutch oven, brown meat thoroughly. Add water to cover meat by at least 1 inch and add chile broken in pieces. Simmer for 4 or 5 hours adding water as needed. When meat is real tender, allow water to boil down until meat is not quite covered. Salt to taste and serve with warm tortillas.

Note: For a more fiery chile, leave the chile seeds in.

When you breed a beef animal with a buffalo you get a calf called beefalo.

Chapter 12

EQUIPMENT

I assume that most folks reading this book have access to a pretty well supplied kitchen. Therefore, I shall endeavor to point out a few items which I find indispensable in the preparation of a full fat-free menu which you might not have.

Cast Iron Cookware

Non-stick cookware doesn't hold up under the strain of non fat cooking. Cast iron cookware, when seasoned and used in conjunction with a nice strong stainless steel pancake turner, is practically indestructible. Cast iron can be purchased at your local discount department stores and is priced quite reasonably.

Often times when preparing meats that need to be floured and then browned, it is crucial not to burn the drippings and flour. For example, a fricassee, a ragout (Ra-goo), soups, stews, and many cajun dishes require a well-browned flour for color and seared meat for flavor. This can be accomplished easily in cast iron cookware. Depending on the number of people you are cooking for, I would recommend a selection from the following:

Small dutch oven with top,
10 inch diameter x 4 inches deep
Large dutch oven with top,
13 inch diameter x 5 inches deep
Large skillet,
12 inch diameter x 2 1/2 inch deep
Medium skillet,
10 inch diameter x 2 inch deep
Small skillet, 7 inch diameter x 2 inches deep

Griddle, 10 inch diameter

By the way, a dutch oven is just a cast iron pot with a lid. It can be placed close to an open fire for baking bread or simmering a hearty stew. I use the large Dutch oven in preparing whole turkeys with stuffing and for big family get togethers.

To season your cast iron cookware, just coat lightly with vegetable oil and bake the pans empty at 300 degrees F for an hour. Don't put oil on the outside of the pans when seasoning. This procedure results in a non-stick coating closely resembling commercial non-stick cookware. The big difference is that if you scratch the coating on your seasoned pan, you can always re-season it by coating lightly with oil and baking it again.

These are tips on cast iron cookware maintenance. First, don't wash it in an automatic dishwasher. Secondly, don't allow real acidic foods like tomatoes to stand very long in the cast iron pot. Thirdly, never put your cast iron cookware away while it is wet as it will rust. Cast iron pots always add minute amounts of dietary iron to your food. This is considered an advantage for those folks who need extra iron.

Stainless Steel Whisk

A 12-inch whisk is regularly used to blend flour, used as a thickening ingredient, and liquid. Since we no longer make a roux in the traditional sense of adding flour to grease, we now must mix our flour in another liquid. These liquids can be water, milk, broth, or other mediums. After the flour is mixed in a bowl with a whisk, it generally is then added to whatever we wish to thicken.

Egg whites can be quickly broken down into a liquid with a quick whisking.

STAINLESS STEEL PANCAKE TURNER
Invaluable in preparing hash browns, burgers, pancakes, etc.

STAINLESS STEEL SKEWERS
You should get to know "kebobs" if you are not already acquainted with them.

PORTABLE ELECTRIC HAND MIXER
You need a mixer of some sort. An inexpensive hand mixer works well with a minimum of clean up and storage time.

SPRING FORM PAN
If you don't make cakes, you won't need this, but if you want an occasional cheesecake (page 303) you will.

STAINLESS STEEL MIXING PANS
If you are going to make bread, you need mixing pans. I recommend a set of 3 measuring in diameters of 10 inches, 13 inches, and 16 inches. When making bread for two, I generally use the 13 inch pan and do the kneading right in the pan. I don't like to clean up a floured board or counter top if I don't have to.

Chapter 13
No Fat Quick Cooking

O̲ne-half the time spent being a cook is used up in cleaning pots, pans and the kitchen in general. This chapter will help you eliminate a lot of clean-up and some preparation time.

The basic idea is to prepare a complete meal in the skillet or dutch oven which not only cooks all the ingredients but doubles as a serving dish also. Electric crock type cooking has been well expounded on in other books and is an excellent cooking method for soups, stews and beans.

I'll give you a few examples and then you can let your imagination create those meals that appeal to you.

FISH FILETS, BROCCOLI & GOLDEN SAUTE™
For 2

In large skillet bring water required for 1 package of Lipton® Golden Saute™ to a boil. Add dry ingredients, place fish filets on top and broccoli florets around edges. Cover and simmer until fish flakes. Sprinkle fish with paprika, place skillet in center of dining table and enjoy.

BLACKENED FILETS, CAJUN RICE & KALE
For 2

In medium veggie sprayed skillet place 2 filets covered with blackening spices. (Filets could be turkey breast, chicken breast, venison, buffalo or beef eye of round) Sear meat, cook until done and remove. In same skillet place water required to cook 1 packet of Lipton® Cajun Rice and add a couple of handfuls of fresh leafy kale or spinach and boil for 5 minutes before adding rice. Push greens off to one side and add rice and follow directions. When rice is done place filets on top with a couple thick slices of home made bread, cover and allow to warm. Serve.

BAKED BREAST OF CHICKEN, STUFFING, VEGGIES AND GRAVY

In dutch oven prepare 1 box stuffing mix. Push to one side and place 3 or 4 cups of large cut chunky veggies such as carrots, broccoli, cauliflower, etc. Spoon stuffing on top of veggies and place seasoned chicken on top of stuffing. Add 1 tablespoon flour to 1 can of defatted chicken broth and pour into bottom of pan. Cover and bake in 350 degree F oven for 1 hour. Remove to dining table and serve.

SAUTEED MEAT, RICE, BEANS & YAMS

In medium veggie sprayed skillet brown your choice of tender meat or poultry. Add 1/2 can chicken broth and simmer until meat is done. Remove meat. In same skillet with meat juices prepare 1 packet Lipton® Rice & Beans with sauce. Add a drained can of yams to one area of the skillet and cook until rice is done. Put 2 thick slices of bread on top of rice along with cooked meat, garnish and serve.

MEAT, POTATOES & WHOLE KERNEL CORN

In medium veggie sprayed skillet brown meat (your choice of very lean items) add a chopped small onion and 1/2 can chicken or beef broth. Push meat and onion off to one section of skillet and place 3 medium potatoes cut to bite sizes in skillet add 1 cup water, cover and simmer until potatoes are done. Combine 1 tablespoon flour to 1/2 can broth and pour over potatoes. Continue simmering uncovered until gravy is thickened. Push potatoes together in order to make room for 1 small can of well drained canned corn. Remove from heat, cover and allow corn to warm. Garnish with fresh parsley and serve.

MEAT STEW & DUMPLINGS
For 2

In veggie sprayed dutch oven brown enough meat or poultry cut into bite size pieces for 2 people, add 1 cup water, and a handful each of your favorite frozen veggies. Simmer until tender and add 1 can chicken broth to which has been added 1 tablespoon of flour. Place 1 can of low fat biscuits on top of stew, cover and simmer for 20 minutes. Garnish and serve.

OPEN FACE BARBECUE SANDWICH
For 2

In small veggie sprayed skillet, brown filets of choice. adding a small amount of chicken broth to facilitate browning. Allow broth to cook off leaving a brown residue as meat cooks. Add 1/2 can chicken broth and 2 thick slices of a big onion (break down into onion rings).

Simmer until onion rings are tender and meat is done. Top the filets with 1/4 cup of your favorite barbecue sauce allowing to mix with onions and broth. Uncover and simmer slowly until sauce is thick, remove from heat.

At the table, spoon filets onto 3/4" thick slices of fresh bread and top with onion and barbeque sauce.

I'm sure by now you realize that you are going to have only one pan to clean up. That's nice and it saves time.

Chapter 14
Recipes and Preparations

RECIPE ANALYSIS

The individual analysis of each of over 400 recipes was deemed to be a very redundant exercise. From a logical perspective, if you strictly adhere to the purchasing principles expounded in earlier chapters (*i.e., Buy only products which contain no more than 1 gram of fat per serving or with meat products, no more than 1 gram of fat per ounce.*) then the following recipes should not greatly exceed 1 gram of fat per normal serving.

If you would like to know the calories, fat, saturated fat and other nutrients in any recipe in this book just send your address and $3.00 to cover handling and shipping to:

Gene Millen, Pres.
Vital Life Center
3184 Collins Drive
Merced, CA 95340

I. APPETIZERS

Fat free appetizers can make a positive statement at any function, whether a cozy fire side meal with your mate, the local bridge club, or a corporate Christmas party.

Cold appetizers can be presented on fat free crackers, breads, or as dips. Vegetables such as mushrooms, celery, or cherry tomatoes may be stuffed early in the day, covered with plastic wrap, and refrigerated.

Hot appetizers should be prepared later, towards meal time, and in sufficient volume.

DIPS AND SPREADS

A plate of icy-cold raw vegetables is always appropriate, appreciated, and they won't spoil your appetite.

ONION DIP

Lipton® dehydrated onion soup mix
Sour cream from page 321

Mix and blend quantity to taste.
For more color add chopped green onion tops.

MEXICAN SOUR CREAM DIP

1   cup sour cream from page 321
2/3   cup fat free mayonnaise
1/3   cup your favorite chunky salsa
      or taco sauce
1/2   teaspoon minced garlic
2   tablespoons minced sweet onions
1   tablespoon chopped parsley or cilantro
      Salt & pepper

Mix and season to taste

EASY BEAN DIP (REFRIED BEANS)

Pinto or Black Beans
Taco Seasoning

Mash beans and add Taco Seasoning to taste.

PINTO BEAN AND GREEN CHILE DIP

2	cups mashed pinto beans
1/2	cup chopped green chiles (well drained)
1/4	cup thick & chunky salsa
	or taco sauce (your favorite)

Mix all ingredients thoroughly.
Can be served hot by topping with Fat Free Cheese Singles and warming in oven.

TUNA SPREAD

7	ounce canned tuna in water
1	tablespoon sweet onion
2	tablespoons fat free mayonnaise

Puree tuna and onion in blender add the rest and chill.

MEXICAN SALSA

2 cups your favorite salsa or taco sauce
1 anaheim (green) chile finely diced
1/4 cup finely diced sweet onion

Mix and chill

DEVILED EGGS

1/2   cup Egg Beaters® egg substitute scrambled
4   hard boiled eggs
2   tablespoons fat free mayonnaise
1   tablespoon Dijon mustard
1   tablespoon minced parsley
      Paprika
4   tablespoons pickle relish

Scramble Egg Beaters® and allow to cool. Peel hard boiled eggs and cut in long halves. Discard yolks. Mix in blender scrambled Egg Beaters®, mayonnaise, relish, mustard, and parsley. Fill hard boiled egg halves with mixture and sprinkle lightly with paprika.

SMOKED TURKEY SPREAD

1   cup finely chopped smoked turkey breast
2   tablespoons fat free mayonnaise
2   tablespoons chopped dill pickle

Mix and chill

CLAM DIP

2   cups lite sour cream
6 1/2 ounce can minced clams
1/4   cup fat free mayonnaise
1   tablespoon worcestershire sauce
1   tablespoon grated onion
      dash cayenne pepper

Mix all ingredients and chill.

RANCH DIP

2   cups fat free ranch dressing
1/4   cup finely diced red
      or orange bell pepper

Mix together

ROQUEFORT & HAM DIP

2   cups fat free roquefort dressing
1/4   cup finely minced turkey ham
      dash of cayenne pepper

Mix and chill.

CHICKEN SPREAD

7   ounce canned white chicken meat
      packed in water
1   tablespoon grated sweet onion
1   tablespoon sweet pickle relish
4   tablespoons fat free mayonnaise

Puree chicken in blender, add rest of ingredients and chill.

CREAM CHEESE & MARASCHINO CHERRY SPREAD

1/2   cup cream cheese from page 322
1/4   cup maraschino cherries, minced
1   packet artificial sweetener or sugar

Mix well and serve on warm fresh bread or slice of cake.

CREAM CHEESE & CELERY SPREAD

4	tablespoons celery, finely chopped
1	tablespoon onion, finely chopped
1/4	cup cream cheese from page 322
	paprika

Mix well and sprinkle with paprika.

CREAM CHEESE & PIMENTO SPREAD

1/4	cup cream cheese from page 322
2	tablespoons pimento, finely chopped
	salt and pepper to taste

Mix and serve.

CREAM CHEESE & GREEN CHILE SPREAD

1/4	cup cream cheese from page 322
3	tablespoons anaheim green chile finely chopped

Mix and serve on baked corn tortilla chips

CREAM CHEESE & PICKLE SPREAD

1/4	cup cream cheese from page 322
2	tablespoons pickle, your choice

Mix and serve.

CREAM CHEESE & WATERMELON RIND SPREAD

1/4	cup cream cheese from page 322
3	tablespoons pickled watermelon rind, finely chopped
1	packet artificial sweetener or sugar

ITALIAN TOMATO SAUCE & BREAD STICKS

1	27 1/4 oz. can of Hunt's® Chunky Style Spaghetti Sauce with tomato chunks
1	cup diced green pepper
1	cup diced sweet onion
1	cup diced fresh mushrooms
	loaf bread (homemade preferred but fat free Italian or French will do)

Mix sauce and veggies and simmer until veggies are done.

Slice loaf bread 1 inch thick and then cut each slice into one inch sections forming bread sticks. Sprinkle with Butter Buds® Sprinkles and garlic powder and toast under broiler. Serve beside sauce.

ITALIAN MEAT BALLS

	Italian tomato sauce
1	package ADM Midland Harvest Burger® mix

Reconstitute Burger mix with water; form into meat balls and simmer in sauce for 20 minutes. Serve hot.

ITALIAN MUSHROOMS

Italian tomato sauce
2   cups medium to large mushrooms

Simmer mushrooms in sauce for 20 minutes. Serve hot.

CORNBREAD STUFFED MUSHROOMS

1   pound large stuffing size mushrooms
1   6 oz. package Stove Top® Cornbread Stuffing Mix

Remove stems carefully from mushrooms. Set caps aside. Dice finely the stems and add to 1 1/2 cups water and vegetable seasoning packet in a saucepan. Bring to a boil. Reduce heat and let stand for 5 minutes. Stir in stuffing crumbs. Fluff with fork, then stuff mushroom caps. Place stuffed mushroom caps on cookie sheet and broil for 5 to 8 minutes until tops are lightly browned garnish with parsley and serve hot.

BURRITOS

4   ten-inch fat free flour tortillas page 266
1   pound ADM Midland Harvest Burger® mix
1   packet taco seasoning
1/4   cup chopped tomatoes
1/4   cup chopped green chiles
1/4   cup chopped sweet onions
6 oz.   package fat free mozzarella (grated)

Reconstitute burger mix. Add taco seasoning, green chiles, onions, and tomatoes.

Simmer in skillet for 10 minutes. Spoon mixture onto tortillas, sprinkle with cheese, roll up and wrap with aluminum foil. Place in warm oven to hold till serving time. Platter and allow guest to cut into desired lengths with sharp knife.

NACHOS

1	8 oz. package corn tortillas
2	cups chili con carne page 87 or 199
8	slices Fat Free cheese slices
1/4	cup chopped green chiles
1/4	cup chopped sweet onion
	A dollup of low fat sour cream

Cut each tortilla into six pie shaped sections. Bake at 325 until crisp (about 20 minutes) arrange some tortilla chips on a round serving dish. Spoon on some of the chili con carne and some of the sliced cheese. Top with more chips, green chiles, onions, more chili con carne, and cheese slices. Place under broiler until cheese begins to melt. Remove, garnish with a dollup of sour cream. Sour cream should top the pyramid of chips and other ingredients.

BARBEQUE WIENERS

1	Package Hormel Light & Lean® frankfurters
1	Cup barbeque sauce

Cut frankfurters into bite size prices, add barbeque sauce, heat and serve.

II. SOUPS & SALADS

In Exeter, New Hampshire, you can sit down at a crooked table placed on a slanting, uneven floor at the famous "Loaf and Ladle" restaurant and enjoy hearty homemade soups and thick slabs of homemade bread. When you leave, your tummy smiles and your mind is at peace with the world. You have just satisfied all the basic instincts of the ancestral hunter-gatherer.

In this case all you gathered was enough money to pay for the soup but for those cooks behind the counter, it has been the combining of the things "gathered" and the things successfully "hunted" into a triumphant, simple meal.

Try this one for pure satisfaction; prepare a soup in a dutch oven, cover and set pot next to an open fire (fireplace, campfire, etc.). At meal time, preferable after dark, ladle up bowls of soup and serve with hot fresh sour dough rolls (page 261). I guarantee satisfaction!

SOUPS

BEAN & VEGETABLE SOUP

1 1/2	cups dried pinto beans
2	quarts water
2	cans beef broth, defatted
1/2	cup tomato sauce or
1	cup chopped fresh tomato
1/2	cup chopped carrots
1	cup shredded cabbage
1/2	cup chopped onion
1	chopped medium potato
2	tablespoons chopped parsley (optional)
1	cup chopped kale, spinach, or other green
	Salt and pepper to taste

Wash and soak beans overnight in water. Boil beans until tender, adding more water if necessary. Put in vegetables and cook until done. Season to taste.

BLACK BEAN SOUP

1	pound black beans
1	onion
2	cloves
1	bay leaf
1	teaspoon dry or fresh parsley
1	chopped medium onion
1	chopped green pepper
1	tablespoon minced garlic
1	can defatted chicken broth page 125
1	teaspoon oregano
1	teaspoon sugar
1	teaspoon vinegar
1	8 oz. can tomato sauce
1/2	cup red wine
	Chopped green onion tops

Clean and soak beans overnight. Add onion with two cloves stuck into it, bay leaf, parsley, and boil until tender. In skillet, cook chopped onion, green pepper, and garlic in chicken broth. Add to beans and cook until thickened. Pour in red wine and simmer for 5 minutes. Garnish with chopped green onion tops.

CREAM OF MUSHROOM SOUP

1	pound fresh sliced mushrooms
1	can defatted chicken broth page 125
2	cups evaporated skim milk
1/2	medium chopped onion
1	tablespoon parsley flakes

1   tablespoon flour
1   tablespoon red wine
        Salt and pepper to taste

In sauce pan, saute mushrooms and onions in chicken broth. Add parsley and red wine. Combine milk and flour thoroughly and add to mushrooms. Simmer to thicken and season to taste. For thinner soup, add more skim milk.

MEXICAN CHICKEN SOUP

2   boneless, skinless chicken breasts
1   can defatted chicken broth page 125
1   cup water
1   cup mexican style stewed tomatoes or
        tomatoes and green chiles
2   fresh chopped anaheim green chiles
1   medium chopped onion
2   cups or 1 can drained pinto beans
        Salt and pepper to taste

Dice chicken into bite size pieces and simmer in large sauce pan with chicken broth until tender. Add other ingredients and simmer until onions and peppers are tender. Season to taste. Serve with tortillas.

CHICKEN NOODLE SOUP

4   cans defatted chicken broth page 125
1   stalk celery
1/4   cup diced onions
2   ounces dry pasta (your choice, but no
        egg noodles)
3 1/2   ounces canned white chicken in water
2   tablespoons chopped parsley
        Salt and pepper

Simmer broth, celery and onions 5 to 7 minutes. Add pasta and cook until tender. Add chicken and salt & pepper to taste.

CHICKEN DUMPLING SOUP

Prepare chicken noodle soup but replace pasta with spoonfuls of vegetable cobbler dough page 285. Simmer until dumplings are done.

VEGETABLE BEEF SOUP

6 oz. defatted roast beef, leftovers, or 6 oz. package deli oven roasted cured beef - 98% fat free

4	cans defatted beef broth page 125
2	scraped and sliced carrots
	Leftover vegetables such as string beans, corn, peas, etc.
1	small bunch of fresh greens (kale, spinach, etc.)
1	small zucchini or yellow squash
1	cup chopped onions
	Salt and pepper to taste

Add all ingredients and simmer until carrots are done. Season with salt and pepper after cooking.

Note: for beef barley soup add 3 tablespoons barley and cook until tender (about 45 minutes).

NAVY BEAN SOUP

2	cups dried navy beans
	water to process
1	large diced onion

1	slice stalk celery
1	teaspoon Molly McButter® bacon flavor sprinkles
4	slices cubed turkey ham - 96% fat free
	Salt and pepper to taste

Soak beans overnight; add water to make 2 quarts in soup pot. Add all ingredients except salt & pepper and simmer for 3 to 4 hours until beans are soft. Add more water to replace any that evaporates. Remove 3 cups of beans from pot and place in blender; reduce to liquid and put back into soup. Salt and pepper to taste.

SEAFOOD CHOWDER

3	medium sliced potatoes
1	large diced onion
1	teaspoon Molly Mcbutter® bacon flavor sprinkles
1	3 1/2 oz. can minced clams
1	3 1/2 oz. can crab meat
2	pounds frozen or fresh cod fish
1	can evaporated non fat milk
1	teaspoon Butter Buds® butter flavor sprinkles
2	slices diced turkey ham
1	can defatted chicken broth page 125
1	cup water
	Salt and pepper to taste

In soup pot, combine potatoes, onion, clams, crab meat, turkey ham, chicken broth, and water. Simmer until potatoes are almost done then add fish and cook until fish and potatoes are done. Add milk but do not boil. Salt and pepper to taste.

NEW ENGLAND CLAM CHOWDER

4   cups strained chowder clams (reserve juice and add water to make 2 cups)
3   slices turkey ham - 96% fat free
1   medium chopped onion
3   peeled and diced potatoes
3   cups non fat milk
1   tablespoon Butter Buds® butter flavor sprinkles
3   tablespoons flour
     Salt & pepper to taste
     Dash of paprika

Combine clams and juice, ham, onion, and potatoes in soup pot and simmer until potatoes are done. In a bowl, combine milk, butter flavor sprinkles, and flour. Use a whisk or mixer to thoroughly blend flour into mixture. Add to soup pot and simmer to thicken. Sprinkle paprika on each bowl of chowder.

SALADS

The traditional tossed green salad we leave to your imagination and personal tastes. It is important that you always use fat free dressings with any salad. Oil is a bad no-no, as are avocados. We include some of the hearty salads that are sometimes served as a side dish with a meal instead of being served as a lonely first course. Also included are main course salads.

CHEF'S SALAD FOR TWO

Lettuce or greens of choice
Radishes
Celery

Tomato wedges
3   slices fat free cheese cut into strips
1   slice turkey ham cut into strips
2   slices breast of chicken or turkey lunch
    meat - 98% fat free cut into strips
2   deviled egg halves page 101 (optional)
    Your favorite fat free dressing
    Salt and pepper to taste

SUNDAY SUPPER SALAD
Serves 6 to 8

4   slices turkey bacon, fried crisp and
    fat pressed out
1   teaspoon minced garlic
1   bunch watercress
1/2 pound spinach
1/2 head lettuce
1   head endine
2   stalks chopped celery (not 2 bunches)
5   sliced radishes
3   quartered tomatoes
12 finely diced green onions
2   finely sliced carrots
    Salt and pepper to taste
    Fat free dressing of choice or your own
    homemade fat free dressing

Crumble bacon and add to garlic-rubbed salad bowl. Break cleaned greens with fingers and mix all other ingredients in bowl. Chill before serving.

COLE SLAW WITH CELERY SEEDS

3   cups shredded cabbage
1/2 cup cole slaw dressing page 208
1   tablespoon minced onions (optional)

1   tablespoon chopped pimento
1/2   teaspoon dry mustard
1/2   teaspoon celery seeds
         Salt to taste (optional)

Combine and chill until serving time.
Note: For cole slaw with green peppers, replace celery seeds with 1/2 teaspoon chopped green pepper.

MIXED VEGETABLE SALAD (CANNED)

1   can mixed, drained vegetables
         Fat free mayonnaise to taste

Mix and chill until serving.

MIXED VEGETABLES SALAD (FRESH FROZEN)

1   16 ounce package frozen mixed vegetables
3   tablespoons fat free mayonaise
1   teaspoon dried sweet basil leaves
         Salt and pepper to taste

Cook veggies per directions and drain. Combine with mayonaise, basil, salt and pepper. Mix well and chill before serving.

Note: Instead of mayonaise try your favorite fat free salad dressing, also try marjarom or rosemary instead of basil.

WALDORF SALAD

2   cups unpeeled, sliced apples
1   cup diced celery
1/2   cup raisins
1/2   cup seedless grapes

1	teaspoon lemon juice
1	packet artificial sweetener (or sugar)
1/2	cup cream cheese from page 322
	or 1/4 cup nonfat yogurt

Mix and serve.

DILLED SHRIMP SALAD

1	pound shrimp, cooked, cleaned, and deveined
1	tablespoon minced onion
1/2	cup sliced water chestnuts
2	tablespoon creamy Italian salad dressing, fat free
	Tomato wedges
	Sliced mushroom
	Lettuce leaves

Toss shrimp with onion, water chestnuts, and salad dressing. Serve with tomato wedges and mushroom slices on lettuce leaves.

BEET AND ONION SALAD

1	can sliced beets
1	medium sliced onion
1/2	cup vinegar
1	packet artificial sweetener (or sugar) to taste

Combine and chill in refrigerator at least an hour before serving. A real hot weather dish.

TUNA SALAD

Crab may be used instead of tuna but never salmon.

1	7 oz. can tuna in water well drained
1/4	cup chopped celery
1	tablespoon your favorite chopped pickle
1	tablespoon fresh lemon juice
1	tablespoon fat free mayonnaise
	minced parsley

Combine well; may be served on crisp lettuce leaves, shredded lettuce, or stuffing in tomato or green pepper or as a sandwich. Garnish with minced parsley.

CHICKEN SALAD

2	cups white meat chicken cooked, defatted, and sized to choice
1/4	cup diced celery
1/4	cup diced tomato
3	tablespoons fat free mayonnaise
	Salt and pepper to taste

Combine ingredients, adding more mayonnaise if desired. Season to taste. Serve on crackers, toast points, as a sandwich, or stuffing for tomatoes, peppers, or mushrooms. Chopped onions are optional.

CARROT SALAD

2	cups shredded carrots
	Coleslaw dressing page 208
1/4	cup raisins

In mixing bowl, add carrots, raisins, and coleslaw dressing to taste. Cover and chill.

WILTED GREENS & BACON SALAD

One large skillet of your favorite greens (spinach, kale, collards, etc.)
4   strips turkey bacon
1   teaspoon Molly McButter® bacon flavor sprinkles
Water sufficient to wilt greens in skillet (approx. 1/4 cup)

Cook bacon until crispy remove and press with paper towels. Remove all grease from skillet. Wilt greens and drain off all water, sprinkle with bacon flavor, add crisp bacon broken into bite sizes and toss. Serve with red wine vinegar.

PASTA & VEGGIE SALAD

2   cups cooked and drained pasta of your choice
1   cup mixed steamed veggies
Fat free ranch dressing

Mix pasta and veggies. Add dressing to taste.

RICE & WHATEVER SALAD

3   cups cooked rice
3 oz.   turkey ham cut into small strips
1/2   cup uncooked frozen green peas
3   tablespoons chopped green onion tops
1   tablespoon chopped parsley
1   teaspoon mustard
1   tablespoon red wine vinegar
        Salt and pepper
1   cup your imagination

Mix ingredients. 1 cup your imagination might be shrimp, lobster, clams, crab, zucchini, tomatoes, or peppers.

POTATO SALAD

4	cups diced baked potatoes (boiled is OK)
4	tablespoons fat free mayonnaise
2	tablespoons yellow prepared mustard
2	tablespoons sweet pickle relish
1/4	cup diced celery
	Salt and pepper

Mix and add more ingredients to taste if desired.

SEAFOOD SALAD

2	cups cooked seafood of your choice (no fat fish)
2	tablespoons fat free mayonnaise
1	teaspoon capers
2	tablespoons lemon juice
2	tablespoons diced dill pickle
1/4	cup finely diced celery
1/4	cup diced red bell pepper
	Salt and pepper
	Dash of cayenne pepper

Mix ingredients and balance to your taste.

COMBINATION FRESH FRUIT SALAD

2	cups mixed fresh friut of your choice in bite sizes
1	tablespoon fat free mayonnaise
2	tablespoons vanilla fat free frozen yogurt

Mix, cover, and chill. Toss just before serving. Garnish with Grape Nuts® and a sprig of fresh mint.

FRUIT & JELL-0® PARFAIT SALAD

2   packages peach Jell-O® gelatin
2   cups fresh, chopped peach slices
         (canned will do)

Prepare two mixing bowls of peach Jell-O® and chill until almost set. Remove from refrigerator and beat one bowl with electric mixer for four or five minutes until very foamy. Mix in one cup of peaches. In the other bowl, combine unbeaten bowl of Jell-O® and one cup peaches. In parfait or ice cream soda glasses, spoon in alternate layers of beaten Jell-O® and the unbeaten Jell-O®. Chill until set.

TOMATO & BREAD SALAD

3   cups 1 inch pieces no fat french or italian
         bread, stale is OK
2   tomatoes, cut in bite size pieces
1   teaspoon finely minced garlic
1   tablespoon basil
1   medium sliced onion
1   green pepper, cut into bite size pieces
1   sprig fresh or dried parsley
4   tablespoons red wine vinegar
         Salt and pepper to taste
2   tablespoons mock blue cheese crumbles
         (see next page)

Mix tomatoes, bread, garlic, onion, green pepper, basil, and parsley. Sprinkle with vinegar and toss. Cover and refrigerate for two hours. Garnish top with mock blue cheese crumbles, or cheese flavor sprinkles.

MOCK BLUE CHEESE CRUMBLES

2   wafers melba toast
2   tablespoons fat free blue cheese dressing
1   teaspoon dried parsley

Crumble melba toast and mix in parsley and blue cheese dressing. Spread on wax paper and allow to dry.

III MEAT AND POULTRY

Purchasing

When the decision to eat meat has been made, purchases should be carefully considered.

First consideration should be given to meats or poultry products that fit the "1 gram of fat per ounce" rule.

Breast of turkey, breast of chicken, buffalo and venison are at the top of our list.

Buffalo & venison genetically, biologically can not marble. This means that when you eat a piece of this "lean" meat it is not loaded with a lot of hidden fat. These two are so important to the "red meat" eaters that they are covered separately in chapters 10 and 11. Please refer to those chapters for cooking instructions.

BEEF OR LAMB:

Buy only whole roasts that appear very lean. Some grocers market them as "Lite" or "Lean" or similar language. Eye of the round is a good cut. If ground beef is desired, have your butcher grind your roast selection. He'll be glad to. DO NOT purchase ground beef to which SEAWEED and water have been added, unless meat appears very, very lean.

PORK:

Again, buy only roasts, preferably the fresh ham or loin, and have your butcher trim it. It should appear as 100% lean pork.

POULTRY:

On a day-to-day basis restrict purchases to only breast meat. For special occasions buy the whole bird.

LUNCHMEAT:

Labels that read "98% or 99% Lean" produced by a reputable company are acceptable. They include turkey and chicken breast products, some hams, and some beef items.

BACON:

Buy only turkey bacon. Most brands are labeled 2 grams of fat per slice. When cooked crisp and toweled dry only about 1/2 gram of fat remains.

MEAT SUBSTITUTES:

Purchase ADM Midland Harvest Burgers® from a company called Harvest Direct. The telephone number is 1-800-835-2867. This excellent product is available in some stores. Also purchase a small bag of textured vegetable protein from your local health food or specialty store. Also called TVP® or order it from Harvest direct also. More about this product in Chapter 9.

Primary Defatting Process

This process applies to all meats and poultry products. It can be done in the oven or on top of the stove. As an example, let's prepare a pork or beef roast.

Place roast and 1/2 inch of water in oven proof cookware. A cast iron pot with a lid is preferred. Roast meat in 400 degree oven for approximately 20 minutes per pound. Cover roast with boiling water and continue in oven for an additional 30 minutes. Remove and allow to cool on top of stove. Make sure roast is completely covered with water. Place in refrigerator and chill overnight.

Next day skim off congealed fat on top of liquid and remove roast. Boil stock to reduce to good flavor, add bullion if necessary. Thicken gravy. Season to taste. Warm roast in gravy. Serve with mashed potatoes.

When we purchased our beef roast there was no visible fat. Meat packers say that when no fat shows the product is at least 5% fat. This means that in a quarter pound serving there was originally about 6 grams of fat. We have baked the roast and rendered (removed) a portion of the fat, but not all. If cooked well done we have removed about half the fat which means a 1/4 pound serving now has about 3 grams of fat.

For ground beef patties, place in skillet and fry to well done. Cover with water and boil for 30 minutes. Cool and stack patties in container and cover with broth. Refrigerate until fat is solidly congealed on top of liquid. To serve remove patties from broth, wash under the sink faucet and fry again. Use a small amount of water in skillet during reheating. Sprinkle patties with beef bullion powder to increase flavor. Season & serve.

A quarter pound patty started with at least 6 grams of fat and now has a lot less. How much less depends on how thoroughly you cook the patty. A rare or medium rare patty hasn't lost much fat.

Secondary Defatting Process

This process simply repeats the first process on top of the stove and does not require a cooling and congealing step. It primarily applies to left over meat, but could be used for all meat if desired. As an example, let's make shredded beef for Mexican Tacos (page 215).

Slice left over roast beef into thin 1/2 inch strips. Place in sauce pan, cover with water and boil rapidly for 1 hour. Don't run out of water! Pour water off and discard. With two forks shred beef.

Add your favorite salsa and bullion (either beef or vegetable or both). Add chopped onions and peppers and heat until onions are done, being careful to add water to keep mixture from burning.

We have, with this second process, removed most of the fat and some flavor. With the addition of the bullion we put the flavor back in. When this mixture is placed on a crisp baked corn tortilla and then topped with a thin slice of fresh tomato, mozzarella cheese, and sliced jalapeno peppers it fairly burst with rich and exotic flavors. But essentially no fat!

Although these two examples use beef, the same processes apply to pork, lamb, chicken and turkey dark meat. Skinless breast of chicken and turkey may be used fresh if desired; however these two defatting processes will remove fat.

Beef & Chicken Broth Defatting Process

Store canned broths in refrigerator at least overnight before using. After opening with can opener remove congealed fat on top of broth. Some beef broth is already fat free and therefore requires no refrigeration or defatting.

MEAT RECIPES

SMOTHERED BEEFSTEAK

2 lbs. Cooked defatted beef cut 1" thick
2   Tablespoons garlic
2   Large onions
1   Can beef broth

In heavy skillet (cast iron preferred) place 1/4 inch of water and two large sliced onions. Sprinkle with 1/4 cup beef broth and pepper to taste. Place 1 inch thick defatted cooked beef cuts on top of onions. Spread 1 tablespoon garlic (per pound) on top of beef. Cover and simmer gently for 1 1/2 hours. Remove beef cuts to serving dish. To remaining defatted beef broth add two tablespoons flour and mix thoroughly. Add to onions, stir and thicken. Spoon onions and gravy on top of beef cuts. Serve. If desired pack skillet around meat with whole mushrooms.

RED WINE FLAVORED STEW

2 lbs. Beef or Buffalo (very lean roast)
       cut into large pieces

1   Cup red wine
1   Medium onion quartered
1   Carrot cut in half
1   Teaspoon garlic, chopped
1   Small piece orange peel
1   Clove
1/2   Small bay leaf
1/4   Teaspoon thyme
1   Small Tomato, chopped
1   Teaspoon bacon flavoring
1   Tablespoon flour
        Salt and pepper to taste when done

Combine all ingredients (except salt and pepper) in a slow crock cooker and allow to marinate overnight. Next morning set cooker to "low" and allow to cook all day. Remove meat chunks, skim off any fat and strain the juice if desired. Just remove the orange peel and bay leaf, season to taste and serve over elbow macaroni.

CAJUN GREAT FILETS
FOR 2

2   Venison filets regular size or 4 small ones
3   Green onions or 1 small regular onion, sliced
1   Teaspoon garlic, minced
        Cajun blackening spices, (your favorite)
        Flour
1/4   Cup chicken stock, defatted
        Vegetable spray

In veggie sprayed skillet on medium high heat brown onions and garlic. Season filets with blackening spice and dust each filet with flour. Push onions off to the side and brown filets. Pour some of this chicken stock on onions and around filets. Turn filets as browned and continue adding chicken broth in order to brown and cook meat. Serve with salad, parsley buttered rice page 171, and warm bread.

GOURMET BARBECUE TENDERLOIN OF VENISON OR BUFFALO FOR 2

1/2	Pound meat sliced 1/4 inch thick
1/2	Cup chicken broth
1/4	Large onion, sliced thick
1	Cup sweet barbecue sauce

Sour dough bread sliced 1 inch thick. (Sour dough oatmeal raisin page 263 works wonderfully)

Brown meat in skillet, add onions, broth and cover. Simmer until onions are tender. Add barbecue sauce, cover and lower temperature to very low. Let meat sit for 5 or more minutes. Spoon meat onto slices of bread, top with onions and sauce.

HUNGARIAN MEAT & POTATOES

4	Ounces (1/4 pound) diced lean pork, chicken or turkey breast (skinless)
2	Cans chicken broth (defatted)
1	Medium onion, chopped
2 lbs	Potatoes, peeled and sliced
1/8	Teaspoon black or white pepper
1	Teaspoon sweet Hungarian paprika
2	Tablespoons flour

In cast iron dutch oven or skillet brown meat and flour adding enough chicken broth to keep from burning.

When meat and flour is well browned add rest of the ingredients and simmer uncovered until potatoes are tender.

This is an excellent "left-over", as the flavors mingle and the dish takes on it's own identity.

POT ROAST BEEF SOUP & SANDWICH

1	Pound eye of round roast beef & broth defatted page 123
	Water to process
2	Bay leaves
1	Large tomato peeled & diced
1/2	Cup whole kernel corn
1/2	Cup okra, frozen
1/2	Cup green peas, frozen
2	Medium potatoes, peeled & quartered
1	Cup greens, chopped
1/4	Cup leftover beans
3	Medium carrots, cut in 2 inch chunks
1	Can beef broth, defatted
1	Medium onion, diced
1/2	Stalk celery, chopped
	Salt & pepper to taste

In heavy kettle or dutch oven combine beef, beef broth, bay leaves, onion, carrot, celery and tomato. Boil on medium heat for 1 hour, add corn, okra, peas, potatoes, greens, beans and simmer for 30 minutes more or until potatoes are tender. Remove roast beef to cutting board. Correct liquid in soup by adding water or broth. Slice beef and serve on slices of Potato-Oatmeal Bread page 245.

SALISBURY STEAK

1	Packet Midland Harvest Burger® Mix
1	Cup chopped sweet onions
2	Tablespoons dry onion soup mix
1	Can defatted beef broth
1/2	Bell pepper
1 1/2	Tablespoons flour

Reconstitute Burger Mix as per instructions (let sit 15 minutes). Add sweet onions and onion soup and mix thoroughly and form into four patties.

Spray cast iron skillet lightly with veggie spray and brown patties on both sides. Blend broth and flour thoroughly and pour over patties. Lift patties to allow broth to underside. Top with green pepper rings and let simmer for 15 minutes.

Serve over a bed of rice or with mashed potatoes.

CAJUN BEEF

2	Cups shredded beef page 124
1	Can defatted beef broth
1/4	Cup chopped green onions
1	Cup whole fresh mushrooms
1	Tablespoon minced garlic
1	Tablespoon Louisiana Hot Sauce
1/2	Teaspoon paprika
1/2	Cup diced fresh tomatoes
	Cayenne pepper, salt & pepper to taste

In large cast iron skillet combine everything except the mushrooms and beef. Simmer slowly for 1 hour. Add mushrooms and beef and simmer for 30 minutes. Goes great on top of instant white rice.

CREOLE BEEF HASH

1/2	Cup defatted beef broth
2	Cups left over beef
1	Medium to small onion
1	Cup chopped uncooked potatoes
	Dash ground clove
	Salt, pepper and cayenne to taste

Mince beef very fine but do not puree.

Combine all ingredients in heavy skillet and simmer gently for about 30 minutes until potatoes are done. Add hot water if necessary to maintain simmer.

BEEF POT ROAST

3	or 4 lb. Beef roast
1	Carrot sliced
1	Turnip diced
1	Stalk celery sliced
6	Medium potatoes peeled & halved
1	Can defatted beef broth
2	Tablespoons flour
1	Tablespoon chopped parsley
1	Bay leaf
3	Cups water

In a heavy cast iron pot or dutch oven place roast on top of carrots, turnips and celery. Add parsley, water & bay leaf. Cover and heat on medium-high burner for three hours. During last 1/2 hour cover mixture completely with boiling water and add potatoes. Remove from heat and allow to cool. Refrigerate overnight.

Next day remove congealed fat & discard. Remove roast and potatoes from pot. Reduce liquid to a tasty broth by boiling. Mix flour and defatted canned beef broth thoroughly and add to boiling stock. Thicken, add roast and potatoes to reheat. Simmer until roast is hot. Serve.

BEEF STROGANOFF

2	Cups defatted roast beef page 123, sliced thin, 1 inch wide
1	Tablespoon minced onion
1	Tablespoon Butter Buds® Butter Flavor Sprinkles
1	Cup sliced fresh mushrooms
1/2	Cup light sour cream
1/2	Cup defatted beef broth
	Dash of nutmeg
	Salt & pepper to taste

In heavy skillet add onions and beef broth; boil for 3 or 4 minutes add beef, Butter Buds® and mushrooms, and simmer for 5 minutes. Add nutmeg and salt & pepper to taste. Add sour cream but do not allow to boil. Serve immediately.

GRILLADES
(Fried Beef Steak or Fricasee)

	Eye of the round roast, thinly sliced
1	Can defatted beef broth
	Flour
	Cayenne, salt & pepper to taste

Slice beef as thin as possible, pepper to taste. Flour each steak on both sides. In cast iron skillet spray lightly with butter flavored veggie spray. Heat skillet to medium -high temperature. Have the beef broth on top of stove next to skillet with a tablespoon. Place steaks in hot skillet. After 1 minute lift each steak with pancake turner and put one tablespoon of the beef broth under each steak. Put several tablespoons of beef broth around perimeter of the skillet. Turn steaks over and repeat process. When done remove steaks.

NOTE: Pork, venison, buffalo or poultry can also be prepared like this.

GRILLADES WITH GRAVY
(Fried Beef Steak with Gravy)

Prepare steaks as in preceding recipe, leaving sauce in skillet.

Gravy

1	Tomato, diced
1	Medium onion, chopped
1	Teaspoon minced garlic
	Remaining beef broth or 1 cup water
1	Tablespoon flour
1	Teaspoon Louisiana Hot Sauce

To sauce already in skillet add the onions, tomatoes, garlic and hot sauce and simmer until onions are done. To left over beef broth add the flour and mix thoroughly then add to skillet and thicken the gravy simmering for 2 or 3 minutes. Remove and serve.

PORK STEAK & ROASTS

Prepare pork as you would beef page 123 through page 125 substituting chicken broth for the beef broth.

PORK STEAK AND SWEET POTATOES

2	Sweet potatoes, peeled & sliced
8	ozs. thinly sliced pork
2	Tablespoons flour
	Salt & pepper to taste
1/2	Cup water

Boil sweet potatoes for 20 minutes, drain and set aside. Prepare pork as for Fried Beef Steak Page 131 using defatted chicken broth. When steaks are done remove. Combine 1/2 cup water & flour, mix thoroughly add to skillet and stir well to make gravy. Add sweet potatoes and place steaks on top. Simmer briefly to reheat steaks and serve from skillet.

POLISH PORK & KRAUT

Same recipe as for Pork Steak and Sweet Potatoes substituting:

1	Cup shredded cabbage and
1	Cup sauerkraut for the sweet potatoes - omit gravy

SWEET AND SOUR PORK

1 lb	Defatted roast pork page 123
1/2	Cup soy sauce
2	Bell peppers sliced
1	Medium onion quartered

1	Cup pineapple chunks
1	Cup sweet & sour sauce
1/4	Cup defatted chicken broth

Marinate pork slices in soy sauce for an hour or so, turning meat several times. In hot skillet add chicken broth, peppers and onions boil vigorously for one minute stirring constantly. Remove from skillet. Drain pork and add to skillet along with pineapple, bring to boil and simmer 3 minutes. Add peppers, onions and sweet & sour sauce. Simmer for 1 minute. Serve with steamed rice.

HUNGARIAN PORK & EGG NOODLES

4-6 oz	Lean pork, all fat trimmed, & chopped
1	Cup onions, chopped
2	Cans defatted chicken broth
1/8	Teaspoon black pepper
2	Tablespoons flour
1	Teaspoon paprika (sweet Hungarian)
6 oz	"No Yoke" egg noodles

In dutch oven brown pork with flour, add broth from time to time as needed to keep from burning. Add the rest of broth and other ingredients and cook until onions are done.

Cook noodles according to directions and add to pork mixture. Remove from heat and allow to sit for an hour or so if possible.

BAUDINS

Baudins were originally a Cajun or Creole blood sausage. Government controls have virtually eliminated this use of blood in sausage making. Modern recipes have added rice and green onions. Instead of stuffing the meat in animal casings this recipe calls for the making of sausage patties. Original recipes called for the mixture to be "seasoned highly" with cayenne and black pepper. Use your own judgement when it comes to the use of very hot cayenne pepper, as it can always be added later.

This sausage when used as a base flavoring agent in Gumbos, Jambalayas and other Cajun or Creole dishes adds a very distinctive flavor and texture.

HOT BAUDIN PATTIES

1	lb ground buffalo (lean)
1	lb turkey sausage
1	lb packet ADM Midland Harvest Burger® mix
1	Cup green onion tops, chopped
1	Teaspoon parsley, chopped
1	Teaspoon garlic
1/2	Teaspoon each of finely ground
	Allspice
	Sage
	Thyme
	Nutmeg
1	Bay leaf
2	Cups water
	Salt, pepper, cayenne pepper to taste
1/2	Cup cooked rice
1/2	Cup beef broth, defatted
	Vegetable spray

In 2 cups water simmer turkey sausage, buffalo, and bay leaf for 30 minutes. Remove from heat and chill. Remove congealed fat. In mixing bowl add onions, garlic, parsley, rice and spices. Mix spices thoroughly. Add turkey sausage along with its broth, the rice, and the beef broth. Add Burger Mix and mix thoroughly. Allow to sit for 15 minutes. Form into patties and fry in veggie sprayed skillet. Freeze and store excess patties to be used in Cajun or Creole recipes calling for sausage.

BREAKFAST SAUSAGE PATTIES

1	lb. fresh ground buffalo (lean)
1	lb. turkey sausage, defatted as in previous recipe
1	lb. packet Midland Harvest Burger® Mix
1/2	Teaspoon onion powder
1	Teaspoon ground sage
1/4	Teaspoon black pepper
1 1/4	Cup broth from defatting the sausage (if necessary add beef broth to make 1 1/4 cup)
1/8	Teaspoon salt
1/8	Teaspoon cayenne

In mixing bowl mix all ingredients thoroughly; let sit for 15 minutes. Form into patties and fry. Freeze excess patties and use for sausage gravy, etc.

HOLIDAY ROAST CHICKEN OR TURKEY & STUFFING

Prepared the day before

Bird or birds, not self-basting or basted
Chicken broth
Salt & pepper to taste
Stuffing page 144 through page 147
Hot boiling water

Remove skin from bird, rub with salt & pepper, and place in cast iron dutch oven. Make sure there is enough room on top to facilitate covering with hot water. A large turkey will need to be quartered. Roasting chickens may need to be split. In 325 degree oven, cover and cook about 25 minutes per pound or until meat thermometer shows 185 degrees in thigh meat, then cover entire bird with hot boiling water and bake for an additional 15 minutes. Remove to top of stove and allow to cool. Chill overnight, removing congealed fat from top of water next morning.

Remove bird from water. Boil water until reduced to flavorful stock. Remove from heat. Pour stock into a saucepan. Prepare stuffing. Place bird and stuffing back into dutch oven with top on. Place in oven at 325 degrees. Thicken stock with flour. When stuffing is done and turkey is heated remove from oven to top of stove. Serve. In post pilgrim times the large dutch oven would have been placed in the middle of the dining table.

CRISPY CHICKEN FILETS

| 1 | lb. Chicken breast filets |
| | Shake n'Bake® seasoning and coating mixture original recipe for pork |

Follow directions on box.

CHICKEN OR TURKEY ENCHILADAS

1	lb. Shredded defatted breast meat page 124
1	Cup chunky salsa, your favorite
1/4	Cup onion, chopped
1	Tablespoon minced garlic
1	Small can green chilies chopped
1/2	Can defatted chicken broth

6-8   Slices fat free cheese
12   Corn tortillas

In medium skillet on medium-high heat add onion, garlic and 1/2 can chicken broth. Simmer for 3 minutes. Add salsa, green chiles and meat. Simmer for 15 minutes. Remove from heat. Spoon mixture onto corn tortillas and roll up. Place in 8" x 14" baking pan. Pour left over juices on top of rolled tortillas. Top with cheese slices. Bake in 350 degree oven for 25 minutes, or until cheese in bubbly hot and starting to brown.

HUNGARIAN CHICKEN OR TURKEY

1   lb. Breast meat, cubed
1/2   Cup onion, chopped
1   Tablespoon Butter Buds® Butter
       Flavored Sprinkles
1/4   Cup tomato, chopped
1/4   Cup water
1   Can chicken broth
3   Tablespoons flour
1/2   Cup extra light sour cream
2   Tablespoons sweet Hungarian paprika
       Salt to taste

In medium skillet add onion and a little broth. Brown onions carefully and add breast meat. Continue adding a small amount of broth so as to allow meat to brown. When meat is browned, add tomato, paprika and water and simmer on low heat for 30 minutes, uncovered. Mix flour with remaining broth and Butter Buds® and add to skillet. On medium heat simmer for 3 minutes. Turn off heat and add sour cream but do not boil. Serve on your own favorite pasta.

MEXICAN CHICKEN OR TURKEY

Very good & easy

1   lb. Breast meat, cubed
1   Cup salsa or taco sauce, your favorite
1/2   Cup chopped onion
1   Tablespoon minced garlic
2   Long green chilies (anaheim) sliced thin
1   Can defatted chicken broth
1/4   Cup red bell pepper
2   Slices fat free cheese
       Salt & pepper to taste

In large skillet brown breast meat using a little broth. Watch carefully and don't burn. Use medium to high heat. Add salsa, onion, garlic, bell pepper and the rest of the broth. Simmer for 25 minutes. Add green chiles and cheese and stir until cheese is melted. Remove from heat and serve with rice & beans page 197.

CHICKEN OR TURKEY CACCIATORE

1   lb breast meat, cubed
1   Tablespoon flour
1   Cup whole medium-small mushrooms
1   Medium onion chopped
1/4   Cup dry white wine (optional)
1   Cup defatted chicken broth
1   Teaspoon garlic, minced
1   Small can tomato sauce
1   Large fresh tomato, chopped
1/4   Teaspoon allspice
1   Bay leaf
1/4   Teaspoon thyme
       Salt & pepper to taste

In large skillet add breast meat and 2 tablespoons broth. Allow to brown but not burn. Add more broth as needed. When meat is somewhat brown on all sides add flour and allow flour to brown but not burn. When brown, add the rest of the broth, onion, wine, garlic, tomato sauce, tomato, allspice, bay leaf and thyme. Simmer for 15 minutes. Add mushrooms and simmer 15 minutes more. Salt and pepper to taste and remove from heat. If possible, allow to sit for 30 minutes - 1 hour, before serving.

CHICKEN OR TURKEY JAMBALAYA

1	lb. Fresh breast meat, cubed
1	Can defatted chicken broth
2	Slices turkey ham (luncheon meat) cubed
1/2	Bell pepper
1	Large onion, chopped
2	Tablespoons minced garlic
1/4	Cup chopped parsley
1	Bay leaf
1	Teaspoon bacon flavor, Molly McButter®
1/2	Teaspoon thyme
1	14 oz. can diced tomatoes
1	Tablespoon Louisiana Hot Sauce
1	Tablespoon Jalapeno peppers
	Salt, Cayenne & black pepper to taste
1	Cup instant rice (uncooked)

In a large stainless steel skillet (at least 12 inch) place ham and breast meat. Allow to brown but not burn, by adding a tablespoon at a time of broth from time to time and allowing broth to evaporate. Add garlic and continue the browning process, using approximately 1/2 can of broth. When brown enough to suit you, add the rest of broth, bell pepper, onion, parsley, bay leaf, thyme, tomatoes, hot sauce and jalapeno peppers. Simmer for 30 minutes. Season to taste. Add rice, cover and remove from heat. Allow to sit until rice is tender.

CHICKEN OR TURKEY FAJITAS

8	oz. breast, shredded
1/4	Cup salsa, your choice
1	Medium onion, sliced
1/2	Bell pepper, sliced
	Salt & pepper to taste
6	Flour tortillas, fat free or see page 266

In medium skillet add onions, peppers, salsa and turkey. Simmer on medium beat until peppers are tender. Remove from heat and spoon onto tortilla and serve.

CHICKEN STEW & DUMPLINGS

1	Pound chicken breast, cubed
2	Medium potatoes, diced
1	Cup kale (or other greens of choice)
1	Medium onion, chopped
2	Carrots, sliced
1/4	Large turnip (optional) chopped
3	Cans chicken broth, defatted
2	Cups water
	Salt, pepper & chicken bouillon granules to taste
2	Tablespoons flour mixed with 1 cup water
1	Package biscuits, (the cheap ones)
	Paprika

In dutch oven combine the chicken, potatoes, kale, onion, carrots, turnips, chicken broth, 2 cups of water and simmer briskly for 20 minutes. Season to taste and add flour mixture. Stir and place biscuits on top of stew, cover and simmer for another 20 minutes. Correct liquid if necessary. When done sprinkle biscuits with paprika.

Since this is a stew, add whatever vegetables you desire.

QUICK TURKEY OR CHICKEN STEW

1	lb. White meat defatted & cubed
2	Cans chicken broth, defatted
1	Teaspoon garlic, minced
1/4	Teaspoon thyme, dried
2	Tablespoons parsley, fresh
1/8	Teaspoon black pepper
1	Bay leaf
1/2	Cup onions, diced
1	Cup baby carrots, cooked
1	Cup potatoes, cubed & cooked
3	Tablespoons flour
1	Teaspoon lemon juice
1/4	Cup dry white wine (optional)

In large skillet simmer onions, garlic, bay leaf, and 1 can of broth until onions are about tender. Add flour to remaining can of broth and mix thoroughly. Add to skillet along with the rest of the ingredients. Simmer gently for 10 minutes. If gravy is to thick add water. If to thin, mix 1 tablespoon flour to 1/2 cup water and add. Serve with hot crusty french bread.

GLAZED TURKEY HAM WITH RED EYE GRAVY

1	Turkey ham
1	Cup orange marmalade (as needed)

Whole cloves
1   Teaspoon instant coffee
        Water

In a pan that fits the ham add water to cover and bring to boil. Simmer for 45 minutes, making sure ham is totally covered with water. Remove and chill, Spoon off congealed fat from the water and remove ham. Dot ham with whole cloves and spoon on marmalade. Place in 350 degree oven for 30 minutes. Remove.
Boil water to reduce to a good strong broth and add coffee. Red eye gravy isn't usually thickened; however, if desired, thicken with flour or cornstarch.

POPOVER CHICKEN

2   Chicken breast, skinless
        Popover batter, page 265
1   Teaspoon dry parsley
1   Teaspoon chicken bouillon granules
        Salt & pepper to taste

Brown chicken and place in veggie sprayed casserole dish. To popover batter, stir in parsley and chicken bouillon granules. Pour over chicken and place in a 350 degree preheated oven for 50 or 60 minutes until done. Serve with mushroom sauce page 204.

LIVER, ONIONS AND BACON

Chicken liver and beef liver contains about 1.1 grams of fat per ounce; however they are high in cholesterol.

Chicken livers

Flour
Salt & pepper, to taste
Chicken broth, defatted page 125
Turkey bacon, cooked crisp and pressed
with paper towel, then crumbled.
Sliced onions
Vegetable Spray

Flour livers, salt and pepper and brown in veggie sprayed skillet. Turn, continue to brown and add some chicken broth. As broth boils off add some more. When browned, add bacon pieces and onion slices, continue cooking until done. Add more broth to maintain sufficient cooking liquid.

MOM'S OYSTER STUFFING
Makes about 2 quarts

1	Cup turkey or chicken broth (defatted)
1	Cup water
2	Cups chopped onion
1/2	Cup chopped celery
12	Cups non fat bread, cubed
1	8 oz. can oysters
2	Teaspoons poultry seasoning
1/2	Teaspoon salt
1/4	Teaspoon black pepper
1/2	Teaspoon ground sage

Boil water, onions and celery until tender. Remove oysters from can and strain juice through a cloth to remove gritty particles.

In large mixing bowl combine all ingredients. Toss and mix well. If you prefer a more moist stuffing add more broth.

CORNBREAD STUFFING

1/2   Cup turkey or chicken breast,
       chopped (optional)
1/2   Cup onion, chopped
2   Cups cornbread, crumbled
1   Can chicken broth, defatted
2   Tablespoons celery, chopped
1 1/4 Teaspoon poultry seasoning
1/2   Cup Egg Beaters® egg substitue
       Salt & pepper to taste
1/2   Cup water

In skillet simmer turkey, onions, celery & 1/2 can chicken broth until onions are tender. Add cornbread, water, the rest of the chicken broth, sprinkle with poultry seasoning and toss to mix. Add Egg Beaters® and spoon into a veggie sprayed casserole dish. Bake at 350 degrees for 45 minutes.

BACON AND SWEET POTATO STUFFING FOR POULTRY

4   Cups mashed cooked sweet potatoes
8   Slices turkey bacon fried crisp, grease
       removed with paper towel then crumbled
1   Cup water
1   Medium onion, chopped
1   Cup celery, chopped
2   Cups dry bread, crumbled
1   Teaspoon salt
1/4   Teaspoon paprika

Saute onions, celery, salt and crumbled bacon in water until tender. Pour over bread crumbs, add sweet potatoes, sprinkle with paprika and mix well.

BACON-VEGGIE STUFFING

8   Slices turkey bacon, fried crisp and grease
           pressed out with paper towels and crumbled
10   Cups stale bread, broken in small bite
           size pieces.
1   Medium onion
1   Cup greens, chopped, spinach, kale,
           collards, etc.
1   Cup asparagus, chopped or other veggie
2   Teaspoon vegetable bouillon granules
1   Can chicken broth, defatted
1   8oz can oyster pieces and broth
2   Teaspoons poultry seasoning
1   Cup water
           Salt and pepper to taste

In skillet, saute onions, veggies and greens in some of the broth until tender. In large mixing bowl or pan combine all ingredients and mix well. Season to taste. Use as stuffing with meat, fish or fowl cooking until meat is done. If stove top stuffing is desired just boil all ingredients before pouring on top of bread pieces, then mix and serve.

APPLE AND BREAD STUFFING

1/4   Cup chicken broth, defatted
1   Tablespoon onions, finely chopped
1/2   Cup celery, chopped
1   Cup soft bread cubes
2   Cups tart apples, finely chopped
1/2   Teaspoon salt
1/4   Teaspoon paprika

Saute onions and celery in chicken broth until tender, pour over bread cubes and mix with apples, add salt and paprika and mix thoroughly.

Note: add more chicken broth if needed.

CRABMEAT STUFFING

1	61/2 ounce can crabmeat
1/2	Cup Egg Beaters® egg substitute slightly beaten
1/4	Cup chicken broth, defatted
1/2	Cup onion, chopped
3/4	Cup celery, chopped
4	Slices turkey bacon, fried, grease removed with paper towel, then crumbled
1	Cup soft bread cubes
	Salt and pepper to taste

Saute onion, celery, cooked bacon in chicken broth, cook until tender reducing liquid to about 2 tablespoons. Pour over bread cubes then add crabmeat and egg substitutes. Mix well. Bake this stuffing with meat, fish or fowl until eggs are throughly done.

CHESTNUT STUFFING

3	Cups chestnuts boiled until soft
1/4	Cup raisins
1	Tablespoon Butter Buds® flavored granules
1	Teaspoons salt
1/8	Teaspoon pepper
1/4	Cup evaporated skim milk
1	Cup dry bread crumbs
2	Tablespoons parsley, chopped fresh
1/2	Cup celery, chopped

1   Tablespoon onion, finely chopped

Chop chestnuts in food processor until the size of rice then combine with rest of ingredients and mix well. Bake with poultry. Recipe may be doubled or tripled for a big turkey.

IV. FISH AND SHELLFISH

The selections of fish should be limited to varieties having a small amount of fish oil or fat. Some acceptable varieties are:
1. Flounder
2. Haddock
3. Halibut
4. Snapper
5. Sale
6. Cod
7. Tuna
8. Sea bass
9. Scrod

Some high-fat varieties include:
1. Jack mackerel
2. Salmon
3. Herring
4. Cat fish
5. Sardines
6. Canned tuna in oil
7. Trout
8. White fish

Shrimp and crab are low in fat, but shrimp are high in cholesterol. Scallops, on the other hand, are low in fat with less than half the cholesterol of shrimp. Fresh oysters contain about 1/2 gram of fat and 14 milligrams cholesterol per ounce. If you are watching your dietary cholesterol, keep a close watch on shrimp consumption, and make substitutions in your recipes calling for shrimp. If you are not watching cholesterol intake, then shrimp are a nice low-fat food item.

All breaded and prepared seafood, unless it passes the 1 gram of fat per ounce test, should be avoided. Some frozen entrees or dinners that contain only 2 or 3 grams per 8 oz (or more) dinner should be considered.

CRISPY FISH FILLETS

1 lb   raw fish
       Shake n' Bake® seasoning and coating
       mixture original recipe for fish

Follow instructions on box.

SHRIMP ETOUFEE

1   pound uncooked shrimp, peeled and deveined
1/4   cup chicken broth
1/2   cup finely chopped onion
1/4   cup finely chopped celery
1/4   cup finely chopped green pepper
1   tablespoon minced garlic
1/2   tablespoon corn starch
3/4   cup water
1   Teaspoon Butter Buds® butter flavor sprinkles
       Salt, pepper, and cayenne pepper to taste

Split shrimp, season with salt, pepper, and cayenne pepper, and set aside.
Simmer onions, celery, green pepper, garlic, and chicken broth until onions are tender. Dissolve corn starch in water, add butter flavor and add to onions along with shrimp. Simmer for 10 minutes until shrimp are just done. Correct seasoning and serve over cooked rice.

BAKED CRABMEAT AND
SHRIMP FOR SIX

1   medium chopped green pepper
1   medium chopped onion
1/2 cup chopped celery
1   small can (6-7 oz) white crab meat
1   pound cooked, deveined shrimp
1/2 teaspoon salt
1/8 teaspoon black pepper
     dash cayenne pepper
1   teaspoon worcestershire
1   cup fat-free mayonnaise
1/4 cup cornflake crumbs

Preheat oven to 350 degrees F. Except for cornflake crumbs, combine all ingredients and spoon into individual oven-proof cookware. Sprinkle with cornflake crumbs and bake for 30 minutes.

CRISPY SHRIMP

Raw shrimp, deveined and well dried
Shake n' Bake®, seasoning and coating mixture, original recipe for fish

Follow instructions on box for fish.

SHRIMP CREOLE

1   lb. deveined shrimp
1   medium chopped onion
1   cup beef broth
1   teaspoon minced garlic
1   cup diced tomatoes
1   cup chopped okra

2   tablespoons finely diced celery
1   tablespoon flour
1   teaspoon Louisiana Hot Sauce
1/4   teaspoon thyme
1   finely chopped bay leaf
        Salt, pepper, and cayenne to taste

In medium skillet on medium heat add onion, garlic, and flour. Brown but do not burn. Add rest of ingredients except shrimp. Simmer for 20 minutes. Add shrimp. Simmer for 10 minutes and season to taste. Serve with boiled rice.

SHRIMP AND SAUSAGE GUMBO

1   lb. medium deveined shrimp
1/2   lb. smoked turkey sausage, thinly sliced
        (1/8 inch)
1   teaspoon paprika
1/2   cup chopped onion
1/4   cup chopped green pepper
1   cup okra
1   sliced jalapeno pepper
2   tablespoons finely chopped celery
1   tablespoon minced garlic
1   finely chopped bay leaf
1   teaspoon creole seasoning
1/4   teaspoon thyme
1   teaspoon Louisiana Hot Sauce
1   teaspoon Worcestershire sauce
1   bunch chopped green onion tops
1   can chicken broth
1   8 oz can oysters and juice strained
4   cups hot water

In Dutch oven, brown sausage, garlic, and onions (well browned but not burnt). Add green peppers, jalapeno pepper, celery, okra, and paprika. Simmer for 10 minutes. Except for the shrimp, add the rest of ingredients and simmer for 40 minutes. Remove and cool. Then store overnight in refrigerator. Remove congealed fat from top of liquid. Heat to simmer and add shrimp. Simmer for 10 minutes and remove from heat. Serve with hot homemade rolls and hot cooked rice. If a thicker gumbo is desired, use flour or cornstarch to thicken after chilling and removing fat.

BLACKENED SHRIMP

Shrimp, deveined
Blackening spices

Skewer shrimp on wooden or stainless steel skewers. Cover abundantly with blackening spices. In heavy cast iron skillet on high heat, spray lightly with veggie spray and place shrimp. Turn over in 3 minutes and blacken other side for 3 minutes. Do not burn.

BROILED CRAB CAKES

1	lb. Crab meat, lump back fin
4	tablespoons fat free mayonnaise
1/8	teaspoon white pepper

Fold ingredients gently together and spoon into individual oven proof serving dishes. Broil for 10 minutes. Sprinkle with paprika and garnish with chopped parsley if desired.

BAKED FISH FROM MEXICO 3

Cod fillets
Picante sauce (your favorite)
Slices fat-free cheese *or shredded fat-free cheese*
Cook fish first, then add toppings.
In individual oven proof serving dishes, place
pieces of fish. Spoon on liberally picante sauce
and top with cheese. Bake until fish flakes
apart.

CREOLE FISH (OR SHRIMP) AND
MUSHROOMS
IN A WHITE CREAM SAUCE

1	pound raw fish (or shrimp)
3/4	cup chopped green onion
	(about 1 small bunch)
1	tablespoon Butter Buds® butter
	flavor sprinkles
1/2	pound mushrooms sliced to bite size
1	cup white wine
1	cup evaporated skim milk
1 1/2	tablespoons flour
	Salt, pepper, and cayenne pepper to taste

Saute onions and mushrooms in wine for five
minutes. Add fish, and simmer for another five
minutes. Meanwhile, combine milk and flour
and mix thoroughly. Pour into fish and simmer
for 2 or 3 minutes. Season to taste and serve
over rice or pasta.

BAKED FISH IN CREOLE
GRAVY FOR TWO

2	fish filets
2	tablespoons flour

1/2	tablespoon Molly McButter® bacon flavor sprinkles
1	stalk celery
1	green bell pepper
1	medium onion
1	8 oz can tomato sauce
1	cup water
	Salt, pepper, and cayenne to taste

Preheat oven to 350 degrees F. In medium cast iron skillet brown flour to dark brown but not burnt. Add onion, celery, water, bell pepper, bacon flavor, and tomato sauce and simmer until onions are tender. Season to taste. Place fish filets in skillet on top of gravy and bake in oven until fish flakes apart (about 40 minutes). Serve on steamed rice.

Since my favorite fish is the ugly orange roughy, I present more "roughy" recipes than you've ever seen before. Although I specify orange roughy, any similar fish can be substituted.

TERIYAKI ROUGHY FOR TWO

1/4	cup teriyaki sauce
1	tablespoon sugar
2	orange roughy filets

In small skillet, mix teriyaki sauce and sugar and bring to a boil. Place fish in sauce and simmer for 5 minutes, turn fish and simmer until fish flakes apart. Serve with rice.

CRAB STUFFED ROUGHY FOR TWO

1	6 oz can crab meat
1/4	cup green bell pepper diced
1	tablespoon fat-free mayonnaise
1	orange roughy filet cut in half.
	Paprika

Preheat oven to 400 degrees F. Combine crab meat, pepper, and mayonnaise and spoon into two individual oven-proof dishes. Place fish on top, sprinkle with paprika and bake until fish flakes apart (12-15 minutes).

STUFFED ROUGHY
FOR TWO

1	orange roughy filet (enough for 2)
1	box stuffing mix
2	portions vegetable of choice
1	can defatted chicken broth
	Paprika

Preheat oven to 400 degrees F. In a large skillet, add broth, stuffing seasoning, and vegetable and simmer on top burner until tender. Correct the amount of liquid in skillet according to stuffing mix directions. (If stuffing mix calls for 1 2/3 cups of water, just make sure your have 1 2/3 cups of liquid in your skillet by adding water.) Push vegetables off to one side of skillet and add stuffing bread. Place fish on top of stuffing, sprinkle with paprika, and pop into the oven to bake until fish flakes apart (10-12 minutes). Remove and serve in skillet.

GENTLE ROUGHY
FOR TWO

1   orange roughy filet (enough for two)
     White sauce from page 202
1   tablespoon chopped fresh parsley

In a small skillet, place fish and a little water and over medium heat simmer for 5 minutes. Turn fish and pour white sauce over fish. Continue simmering for another 5 minutes or until fish flakes apart. Remove from heat, top with parsley, and serve from the skillet.

DRUNKEN ROUGHY
FOR TWO

1   orange roughy filet (enough for two)
1/2 cup white wine
     White clam sauce from page 203
     Chopped green onion tops or chives

Preheat oven to 400 degrees F. Place fish in an oven proof serving dish pour on the wine. Bake until fish flakes apart (12-15 minutes). Remove, spoon on sauce, and sprinkle with green onion tops. Serve hot.

TEQUILA ROUGHY
FOR TWO   *2 without jalapeños*

1   large orange roughy filet (enough for two)
1   chopped anaheim green pepper
1/2 medium chopped onion
     (green onions are fine)
1   medium chopped tomato
1   very optional chopped jalapeno pepper
     (if you don't like it hot, don't add the

jalapeno pepper)
1   ounce tequila
Salt to taste

In skillet, saute onions with a little water until tender. Add pepper and tomato and simmer for 5 minutes. Add tequila and simmer for another minute or so. Salt to taste and remove from heat. Broil fish in oven proof dish until it flakes apart. Remove and top with pepper/tomato mixture. Serve hot.

BROILED ROUGHY WITH HERBED WHITE BUTTER SAUCE
FOR TWO

1   large orange roughy filet (enough for two)
      Fish base veloute' sauce
1/2   teaspoon chopped chives or
      green onion tops
1/2   teaspoon parsley
1/2   teaspoon tarragon
1   teaspoon butter flavoring

Combine sauce, chives, parsley, tarragon, and butter flavoring. Broil fish until it flakes apart in oven proof serving dish. Remove from oven and top with sauce mixture. Serve hot.

BROILED GARLIC BUTTER ROUGHY
FOR TWO

1   orange roughy filet (enough for two)
1   packet Butter Buds® flavoring prepared
      as per directions
1   teaspoon minced garlic
      Salt and pepper to taste
      Cracker crumbs

Fresh parsley

In oven proof dish or individual dishes, place fish. Mix garlic and butter flavoring and pour over top of fish. Add salt and pepper to taste, top with cracker crumbs, and place under broiler until fish flakes apart. Garnish with fresh parsley and serve.

MUSHROOM ROUGHY
FOR TWO

1   orange roughy filet (enough for two)
       mushroom sauce from page 207
       fresh mushroom caps
1   tablespoon chopped parsley

Simmer fish, mushroom caps, and mushroom sauce in a covered skillet for 5 minutes. Turn fish and sprinkle with parsley and continue simmering until fish flakes apart. Serve in skillet.

CAJUN ROUGHY, VEGGIES, BEANS, AND RICE
FOR TWO

1   packet Lipton® Rice and Beans with Sauce
1   cup cut okra
1   medium chopped tomato
1   cup chopped broccoli
1/2   medium thinly sliced onion
1   orange roughy filet (enough for two)
       Cajun seasoning to taste

Prepare Lipton® Rice and Beans per directions (minus any butter or margarine) in a large cast iron skillet. Add tomato, onion, okra, and broccoli and simmer for 5 minutes. Season orange roughy with cajun spices and place on top of rice and vegetables. Cover and continue cooking until orange roughy flakes apart. Add favorite bread on top of rice, cover and place skillet in center of dining table and enjoy. Goes well with cheddar corn bread.

ORIENTAL ROUGHY
FOR TWO

1/4	cup water
1/2	medium thinly sliced onion
1/2	thinly sliced green bell pepper
1/2	thinly sliced red bell pepper
1/2	teaspoon minced garlic
1	teaspoon parsley
	Salt and pepper to taste
1	box Lipton® Golden Saute™ Oriental Style Orange roughy filets for two
	Snow pea pods for two

In large cast iron skillet, saute onion in water until tender. Add peppers, garlic, parsley, salt, and pepper. Cook for 3 or 4 minutes stirring several times. Remove mixture from skillet and set aside. Prepare Golden Saute™ in skillet and simmer for 5 minutes. Place orange roughy on top and spoon pepper mixture on top of fish. Add pea pods, cover, and continue simmering until fish flakes apart.

BEETLE JUICE ROUGHY
FOR TWO

1	small can whole beets
2	tablespoons vinegar

2   tablespoons sugar
2   tablespoons corn starch
1   orange roughy filet (enough for two)

In medium skillet, combine beets with juice, corn starch, vinegar, and sugar. Bring to boil and place fish in liquid (push beets off to side). Simmer for 5 minutes, turn fish, and simmer until fish flakes apart. Serve with rice.

SCALLOPS

If you have ever seen the Shell Oil symbol, you've seen a scallop shell. In days gone by, the scallop shell was used as a plate to eat out of or a cup from which to drink.

There are two types of scallops available in most large supermarket fish sections. The sea scallop is from the deeper sea and is larger than the bay scallop. Bay scallops are smaller and more tender. Both are prepared in the same manner.

Scallops are very low in fat, about 1/4 gram per ounce and as such, are a welcome variation to our diet.

BROILED SCALLOPS
FOR TWO

      Scallops for two
2   tablespoons white wine
2   teaspoons minced garlic
      Salt and pepper to taste

In each of two individual oven proof serving dishes, place 1/2 of the scallops, 1 tablespoon of white wine, and 1 teaspoon of garlic as well as salt and pepper to taste. Broil close to heating element or flame.

BAKED SCALLOPS
FOR TWO

          Scallops for two
1   teaspoon Butter Buds® butter flavor sprinkles
1   teaspoon minced garlic
1   teaspoon minced green onion tops
1   tablespoon chopped parsley
1   teaspoon lemon juice
          Fat-free cracker crumbs
          Salt and pepper to taste
          Paprika

Preheat oven to 400 degrees F. In each of two individual oven proof serving dishes, place 1/2 of the scallops and 1/2 of butter buds, minced garlic, green onion tops, and lemon juice. Sprinkle tops with cracker crumbs and salt and pepper to taste. Bake 10-12 minutes remove, sprinkle with paprika, and serve.

SAUTEED SCALLOPS WITH DILL
FOR TWO

1/2   pound scallops
1/2   cup defatted chicken broth
1   teaspoon Butter Buds® flavored sprinkles
1   teaspoon chopped onion
1   teaspoon dill
          Dash of tabasco
1   tablespoon white wine
          Pepper to taste

In a medium skillet on medium heat, add chicken broth, Butter Buds®, onions, dill, and tabasco. Reduce liquid to about 4 tablespoons. Add white wine, scallops and toss. Simmer only until scallops are heated through. Do not over cook!

BLACKENED SCALLOPS
FOR TWO

1/2   pound scallops
      Your favorite cajun blackening spices for fish
      Vegetable spray

Place scallops on individual skewers. Dust with cajun blackening spices and place on hot veggie sprayed griddle or skillet. Turn over after 3 or 4 minutes and continue cooking until scallops are heated through. Serve on top of a bed of cajun rice.

CREOLE SCALLOPS
FOR TWO

1/2   pound scallops
1   tablespoon flour
1   can defatted chicken broth
2   tablespoons chopped onion
1   tablespoon minced garlic
1/2   cup chopped tomatoes
1   teaspoon tabasco sauce
      Salt, pepper, and cayenne pepper to taste

In a medium skillet over medium-high heat. Put in the flour and brown while stirring. Add a little chicken broth and allow to cook off and brown. Continue to stir, splashing on a little more broth until liquid is quite brown but not burnt. Add rest of broth, onion, garlic, tomatoes, and tabasco sauce. Simmer until onions are tender and season to taste. Add scallops and bring to a simmer for 5 or 6 minutes until scallops are heated through. Serve over rice.

SEAFOOD MEDLEY IN DILL/TARRAGON SAUCE
FOR TWO

1/2	pound cod (or your choice of fish)
1/2	pound large shrimp, peeled and deveined
1/2	pound scallops
2	tablespoons flour
1/2	cup evaporated skim milk
2	teaspoons Butter Buds® flavor sprinkles
1	tablespoon oyster sauce
2	tablespoons clam sauce
1/8	teaspoon pepper
1/2	teaspoon dry tarragon
1/2	teaspoon dry dill weed
2	tablespoons white wine
1 1/4	cup water

Clean fish, cut into bite size pieces, and along with shrimp, place in a skillet with water, oyster sauce, clam sauce, pepper, tarragon, dill weed, white wine and bring to a slow simmer until shrimp are heated through. Remove fish and shrimp with slotted spoon and set aside. Reduce broth to about one cup. In a separate bowl, combine and mix thoroughly the milk, Butter Buds® flavor sprinkles, and flour. Add the flour/milk mixture to the simmering broth and stir as sauce thickens. Simmer sauce until it is slightly thicker than desired. Add scallops, shrimp, and fish. Barely simmer (don't boil) until scallops are heated through. Remove from heat and serve over pasta or toast.

V. POTATOES, RICE, PASTA & DRIED BEANS

This section is dedicated to four of your staunchest allies. If you replace these carbohydrates in part with protein (as in meat) or fat (as in any kind) then fat loss is slowed or in extremes, is reversed (as in gaining). So load up on these four horsemen and let them carry the day.

1. Potatoes

BAKED POTATOES

Never wrap a potato in aluminum foil. It will steam your potato and you'll miss the truly "baked" flavor and texture.

Heat oven to 450 degrees. Clean potatoes by using a vigorous scrub brush. Apply salt and coarse ground black pepper to potato. Place on oven rack apart from each other. Bake for 1 hour. If thicker crust is desired continue baking for another hour.

FRENCH FRIED POTATOES

Potatoes, peeled and cut to even size
Shake n'Bake® seasoning and coating mixture, original recipe for pork

Preheat oven to 400 degrees. Coat potatoes liberally with coating mixture and place separated on baking sheet. Bake for approximately 30 minutes until potatoes are brown and crisp.

POTATOES AU GRATIN

2	Cups potatoes, sliced
1/2	Medium onion, sliced
1	Can chicken broth, defatted
1	Tablespoon powdered milk
4	Slices fat free cheese
3	Tablespoons flour

Preheat oven to 400 degrees. In casserole dish combine potatoes, onion, 2 slices of broken up cheese. Mix flour, milk & broth thoroughly and pour on casserole and top with 2 slices of cheese. Bake 40 minutes or until potatoes are tender and top is browned.

TWICE BAKED POTATO

1	Large potato, baked
2	Slices fat free cheese
1/8	Teaspoon onion powder
2	Tablespoons evaporated non fat milk
1	Teaspoon chives or green onion tops, minced
2	Teaspoons Butter Buds® Butter Flavoring
	Salt & pepper to taste

Preheat oven to 400 degrees. Split potatoes in long halves. Carefully scoop out potato, being cautious not to tear up potato shell. Set shell aside. Combine other ingredients and mash, DON'T BEAT. Spoon into potato shell and bake for 20 minutes or until brown on top and hot inside.

POTATO SKINS

1	Baked potato (left over)
1	Slice fat free cheese
1/2	Jalapeno pepper, fresh & sliced
1	Tablespoon green onion, chopped
	Bacon flavor to taste
1	Slice tomato, chopped
1	Tablespoon light sour cream

Preheat oven to 400 degrees. Slice potato in half length ways. Scoop out part of the potato and discard. Lay cheese on top of potato then add peppers & onion. Sprinkle with bacon flavor. Heat in oven for 10 minutes. Remove, top with tomatoes and sour cream. Serve hot.

MASHED POTATOES

2	Cups potatoes, fresh cooked or instant cooked
2	Tablespoons non fat milk powder
1	Tablespoon Butter Buds® Butter Flavoring
	Salt & pepper to taste

Combine ingredients and whip if necessary.

2. RICE

It is said brown rice is better than white rice and white rice is better than instant rice. But if you are in a hurry, instant rice is great. Wild rice is not rice at all but is grass seed. As one of the four horsemen carrying your carbohydrate load, rice is deserving of your close attention and HIGH usage.

BOILED RICE

Whether white, brown or instant prepare as per directions.

BAKED CHEESE & RICE WITH YOUR CHOICE VEGETABLE

2   Cups rice, cooked
1   Can chicken broth, defatted
3   Tablespoons flour
6   Slices fat free cheese
1   Cup vegetables, cooked your choice

Preheat oven to 400 degrees. Combine ingredients and spoon into a casserole dish. Bake for 20 minutes.

RICE & LEMON RAISINS

1   Cup instant rice, uncooked
1   Cup water
1/4   Cup maple syrup (Maple flavored)
        Juice of 1/2 lemon
1/2   Cup raisins

In sauce pan bring water, raisins, syrup and lemon juice to boil for 3 minutes. Add rice, cover and remove from heat. Let sit for 5 minutes. Fluff with fork & serve. Goes well with baked poultry.

SPANISH RICE   *good & easy*

2   Cups Instant rice, uncooked
1   Cup chicken broth, defatted
1   Cup canned tomatoes, diced
1   Teaspoon garlic, minced

2	Tablespoons onions, diced
1	Fresh Jalapeno pepper, diced
1/2	Teaspoon paprika
	Salt to taste

In sauce pan bring to boil all ingredients except rice. Boil for 3 minutes. Add rice, cover and remove from heat. Let sit for 5 minutes. Fluff and serve.

PARSLEY BUTTERED RICE

For each cup of finished cooked rice, add 1 teaspoon Butter Buds® flavor granules, 1 teaspoon chopped parsley and salt & pepper to taste add during the cooking process.

DIRTY RICE

2	Chicken livers
1	Can chicken broth, defatted page 125
3	Green onions, finely chopped (tops and all)
1	Teaspoon garlic, minced
1	Tablespoon fresh poultry, chopped
1	Cup instant rice
	Salt and pepper to taste

In sauce pan simmer ingredients (except for rice) until livers are done. Remove livers, chop and return to pan along with rice. Simmer to allow rice to absorb liquid, remove from heat.

SHRIMP FRIED RICE

1	6.7 oz. Package Lipton® Golden Saute™, oriental or beef style
1/2	Cup bean sprouts
1/2	Cup Egg Beaters®, scrambled egg substitute

1/2   Cup green onion tops, sliced
1/4-1/2 lb. Shrimp, peeled & deveined

Prepare Lipton® Saute™ as directed in pan
without butter or margarine. After three
minutes boiling time add shrimp to pan and
continue simmering for 7 minutes or until rice is
tender. Remove from heat and let sit for 5
minutes. Add green onions, Egg Beaters®
(already scrambled) and bean sprouts. Toss
gently and serve.

WILD RICE

Wild rice or Mahnomen, as the Indians call
it, has been harvested in the lakes and
streams of the Great Lakes area since long
before the dawn of written history. It is found in
great abundance in the shallow, cool lakes of
northern Minnesota and the adjacent area of
Canada. Recently, successful wild rice farming
has been developed in the same geographic
areas. Now an increasing farm harvest is
becoming available to supplement the ancient
Indian harvest.

The wild rice produced on the wild rice
paddies is identical and indistinguishable in both
appearance and taste from the lake harvest from
which the paddy seed is derived - if both types
are identically processed. Differences in color
and flavor are a result of processing techniques.

In harvesting the lake crop, a boat or canoe
is poled through the wild rice by one person. A
second person bends the heads of the wild rice
plant over the boat with a flailing stick and
strikes them with another such stick to dislodge
the plump, ripe kernels. The unripe kernels

adhere to the stem until ripe, requiring several trips, some days apart, to complete the harvest.

The wild rice grown in paddies is harvested in the most careful, modern method in order to secure the highest possible yield. The water is released in the late summer allowing sufficient period for the ground to firm and yet not impede the growth of the wild rice plant. Large, efficient grain combines are used to harvest the kernels eliminating as much waste as possible.

Wild rice used to be scarce and expensive, but now it's more available and affordable. You'll enjoy the nutty, toasted flavor, the firm, crunchy bite of this elegant grain. A nutritious, high-fiber carbohydrate with only 70 calories per half-cup serving, it goes with today's smarter, "in style" menus.

A LITTLE MAKES A LOT

1   cup wild rice =
3-4 cups cooked =
6-8 servings!

EASY TO PREPARE. Wash wild rice throroughly, in a medium sauce-pan, cover 1 cup wild rice with 3 to 4 cups water. Add 1 teaspoon salt, if desired. Bring to a boil and simmer. Check it after 45 minutes. If most of the grains have split and the inner, lighter part is visible, it's just right. At this stage, it's got good texture and bite.

It you prefer a softer rice, simply cook it a few moments longer, until most of the grains are puffed and some are curly. (But don't let it get mushy.) Most of the water will be absorbed, and the rest can be drained off.

KEEPS WELL. Dry wild rice keeps for months in a dry, tight container. Plain cooked

wild rice should be drained well and stored air-tight. Refrigerated, it will keep well for a week. Frozen, it will keep for months.
VERSATILE. Wild rice adds a special touch to many recipes.
To make a creamy Wild Rice Soup: Add 2 tablespoons cooked wild rice, for each serving to cream of mushroom soup, page 108
To make a Wild Rice Waldorf Salad: Add cooked wild rice to Waldorf Salad recipe, page 114.
To make a Wild Rice Chicken Salad: Add cooked wild rice to Chicken Salad recipe, page 116.
To make Wild Rice Tabbouli Salad: Substitute cooked wild rice for the bulgar in your favorite Tabbouli recipe.

The preceding information along with following recipes have been provided by the Minnesota Paddy Wild Rice Council, St. Paul, Minnesota. I have modified the recipes by removing fatty ingredients.

WILD RICE SAUTE

4-6	cups cooked Wild Rice
1	large onion, chopped
1/4	lb. fresh mushrooms, sliced
1	large Bell pepper, cut into strips (use half red and half green pepper)
1/2	cup chicken broth
	salt or seasoning salt
1/4	teaspoon garlic salt
	pepper, as desired

Saute the onion, mushrooms and Bell pepper in the chicken broth, adding salt, garlic salt and pepper as desired. Cook only until vegetables are tender, but still crisp. Add the wild rice, stir and when wild rice is heated through, serve. Serves 6 to 8, depending upon the amount of wild rice used.

WILD RICE AU GRATIN

4	cups cooked Wild Rice
2	cups sliced fresh mushrooms, about 1/4 lb.
1/4	cup chicken broth
2	cups grated non fat cheese, about 1/4 lb.
	vegetable spray

Saute the mushrooms in the broth until the mushrooms soften slightly. Toss wild rice with sauteed mushrooms and cheese: spoon into a veggie sprayed 2-qt. casserole. Cover and bake at 325 degrees about 20 minutes. Uncover and bake 10 minutes longer. Serves 4 as a main dish, up to 8 if used as a side dish with meat.

WILD RICE STUFFING
Use with poultry, game, roast or chops

3	cups cooked Wild Rice
4	slices turkey bacon
1/2	cup chicken broth, defatted
1	medium onion, chopped
1/2	lb. mushrooms, sliced
3	ribs celery, chopped
1	teaspoon crushed leaf oregano
1/2	teaspoon crushed leaf sage
2	cups bread crumbs
	salt and pepper, if needed

Fry bacon crisp, remove and press grease from bacon using paper towels. Cut bacon into

1 inch pieces and saute with onions, mushrooms, celery and chicken broth until tender.

Add this to the wild rice, along with the oregano, sage and bread crumbs. Adjust seasonings with salt and pepper if needed. Makes enough stuffing for a 10 to 14 lb. turkey. (If cooking separately, bake, covered, in a buttered casserole at 350 degrees for 30 to 40 minutes. Add more chicken stock, if needed, for moisture.)

WILD RICE ORIENTAL SOUP

1 1/2   cups cooked Wild Rice
8   cups chicken stock seasoned to taste
1   whole chicken breast, skinless, deboned
24   fresh small pea pods
18   carrot curls* or 1/4" diagonal carrot slices
2   teaspoons ginger juice, (press fresh ginger
        pieces through a garlic press)

Poach the chicken breast in stock, remove chicken breast and cool. Cut into julienne strips. Poach pea pods in chicken stock until just tender, about 6 minutes; remove from stock

Poach carrot curls in stock about 1 minute (do not overcook). Remove from stock and let cool; remove picks, being careful to maintain "curls".

Strain chicken stock through cheese cloth until it is clear. Add giner juice to stock and adjust seasonings to taste. Reheat stock to serving temperature.

Meanwhile, arrange wild rice and chicken strips in the bottoms of 6 soup bowls. Place 6 poached pea pods in each bowl and divide the stock between bowls, pouring slowly into the sides of bowls. Arrange 3 carrot curls in the center of each serving and serve immediately. Serves 6, as a first course soup or a light entree.

* TO MAKE CARROT CURLS: Large, thick carrots are best for these. Scrape carrots. With a vegetable parer, cut wide, thin slice down the length of carrot. Roll slice around index finger, fasten with a toothpick.

LEMON-TARRAGON WILD RICE

4	cups cooked Wild Rice
1/4	cup chicken broth
1	tablespoon instant chicken bouillion granules
1	tablespoon fresh lemon juice
1-2	tablespoons chopped fresh tarragon
	salt and pepper to taste
	strips of lemon peel and sprigs of fresh tarragon, for garnish

Mix chicken broth, bouillon granules, lemon juice and tarragon. Cook over low heat until bouillon granules are dissolved, adding a tablespoon of water, only if necessary. Add the wild rice, adjust seasonings if desired, and continue cooking until wild rice is thoroughly heated. Garnish with strips of lemon peel and sprigs of fresh tarragon. Serves 6.

WILD RICE QUICHE FLORENTINE

1 1/2	cups cooked Wild Rice
1/2	cup finely chopped leek
1/4	cup chicken broth (defatted)
1/4	cup finely chopped parsley
1	cup finely chopped fresh spinach, or 1/2 (9 or 10 oz.) pkg. frozen chopped spinach, thawed and drained well
3/4	teaspoon salt

1/4   teaspoon pepper
1/4   cup finely chopped raisens
1   cup Egg Beaters® egg substitute
       (lightly beaten)
1   cup evaporated skim milk
1   (9-inch) pie crust from page 278 (uncooked)
       non-fat plain yogurt or sour cream

Saute the leek in the chicken broth about 2 minutes. Combine this with the wild rice, parsley, spinach, salt and pepper and raisins. Add the egg substitutes and milk and mix well.

Pour the mixture into the pie crust. Bake at 425 degrees for 10 minutes, then reduce heat to 325 degrees and continue baking 30 minutes, or until a knife inserted near center comes out clean. Let set about 15 minutes before slicing. Serve as a main dish with a dollop of yogurt or lite dairy sour cream. Serves 6 to 8.

LOBSTER WILD RICE BISQUE

1   cup chopped onions
1   4 1/2 oz jar sliced mushrooms, drained
2   tablespoons flour
1/2   teaspoon salt
1/2   teaspoon pepper
2   teaspoons crushed rosemary
4   cups chicken broth
1/4   cup cooking sherry
1   cup evaporated skim milk
1   cup chopped tomatoes, fresh or canned
2   cups cooked wild rice
8   ounces Imitation Lobster, cut in 1" chunks
6   ounces yolk free Egg Noodles, cooked
2   cups shredded fat free cheese

Saute onion and mushrooms in 1/4 cup broth. Stir in flour, salt, pepper and rosemary. Cook until bubbly. Gradually add rest of chicken broth, heat until boiling, stirring often. Stir in sherry and milk. Add tomatoes, wild rice, lobster and noodles. Heat thoroughly. Fold in cheese. 8 servings.

TURKEY WILD RICE CHILI

1	medium onion
1	garlic clove, minced
1	pound Turkey Breast Slices, cut in 1/2" pieces
2	cups cooked wild rice
1	15 oz. can great northern white beans, drained
1	11 oz. can white corn, whole kernel
2	4 oz. cans diced green chiles
1	14 1/2 oz. can chicken broth, defatted
1	teaspoon ground cumin
	hot pepper sauce
6	ounces fat free cheese, shredded
	parsley (optional)

Heat 2 tablespoons of chicken broth in large pan over medium heat; add onion and garlic. Cook until tender. Add turkey, wild rice, beans, corn, chiles, rest of broth and cumin. Cover and simmer over low heat 30 minutes or until turkey is tender. To serve, stir hot pepper sauce into chili to taste. Serve with shredded cheese. Garnish with parsley. 6 to 8 servings.

WILD RICE GOURMET BURGERS

4	pounds lean ground buffalo
3	cups cooked wild rice

Mix well. Form into 22 to 24 patties. Freeze in quantities to suit your family. Defrost before pan frying or broiling.

Seasoned burgers - add seasoned salt, minced onion, parsley or other seasonings before freezing.
Cheeseburgers - add a slice of fat free cheese.

WILD RICE LEMON SEAFOOD SALAD

1	cup cooked wild rice
6	Imitation Crabmeat Sticks, cut in 1" pieces
1	cup cooked yolk free egg noodles
1	cup cubed jicama
1	medium avocado, cubed

DRESSING:

3/4	cup lemon yogurt
1/2	cup sour cream (fat free)
1/2	teaspoon curry powder

Lightly toss together salad ingredients. In small bowl, blend dressing ingredients. Top salad with dressing. 4 servings.

ARTICHOKE WILD RICE SALAD

2	cups cooked wild rice
1	cup frozen peas, thawed
1	8 oz. can sliced water chestnuts, drained
1	6 oz. jar marinated artichoke hearts, drained
4	ounces fat free cheese, cubed
1	2 oz. jar diced pimento, drained
6	tablespoons fat free Italian salad dressing

In large bowl, combine salad ingredients and mix with dressing. Chill 4 hours or overnight, to blend flavors. 6 to 8 servings.

DILLY WILD RICE CRABWICH

12	ounces imitation crabmeat, shredded
1	cup fat free cheese, shredded
1/2	teaspoon dill seed
1	cup cooked wild rice
3	ounces cream cheese, softened from page 322
1/2	teaspoon garlic powder
6	drops hot sauce
10	slices french bread, cut in 1/2" slices

Mix first seven ingredients. Set aside.
Spread crab mixture on 5 bread slices. Make a sandwich by topping each with second piece of french bread. Grill until warmed through and browned, about 6 minutes each side. Makes 5 sandwiches.

Variation: Use cocktail rye bread for a grilled mini-sandwich appetizer.

TURKEY WILD RICE MEATBALLS

1	pound ground turkey breast
1	cup cooked wild rice
1/4	cup beef broth (from 15 ounce can)
2	egg whites, slightly beaten
1/4	cup chopped leeks or green onions
1	garlic clove, minced
1/4	teaspoon salt
1/8	teaspoon pepper
	vegetable spray
6	oz. spaghetti, cooked

SAUCE:

1 3/4 cups (or remaining) beef broth
1   6 oz. can tomato paste
1   4 1/2 oz. jar sliced mushrooms, undrained
1/2   cup chopped green pepper
1/4   cup chopped onion
2   tablespoons chopped parsley
       (or 1 tablespoon dried)
2   Tbsp. fresh oregano leaves (or teaspoon dried)

Mix meatball ingredients except for spaghetti. Shape in 1" balls. In veggie sprayed skillet using med.-high heat, brown meatballs; move to side of pan. Add sauce ingredients and carefully stir to blend. Stir sauce and meatballs together. Simmer, covered, about 30 minutes, until sauce is thickened and vegetables are tender. Prepare spaghetti as directed on package. Serve meatballs over spaghetti. 6 servings.
Variation: make smaller meatballs and serve as an appetizer.

WILD RICE TETRAZINI

1   cup chopped green pepper
1   cup chopped onion
1   8 oz. jar sliced mushrooms, drained
1   pound ground turkey breast
1   teaspoon salt
1   teaspoon pepper
2   teaspoons garlic powder
3   tablespoons flour
2   cups chicken broth, defatted
2   cups milk, evaporated, skimmed
1/2   cup cooking sherry

2   cups spagehetti, cooked and drained
3   cups cooked wild rice
2   cups shredded fat free Mozarella cheese
       parsley flakes

Preheat oven to 350 degrees. Saute green pepper, onion and mushrooms in 1/4 cup chicken broth. Add turkey, brown. Add seasonings. Mix flour with remaining broth stir and cook 5 minutes. Add sherry. Heat thoroughly. Place spaghetti and wild rice in a 5 quart veggie sprayed casserole. Mix in 1 cup cheese. Pour turkey mixture in casserole; lightly mix. Top with remaining cheese and parsley. Cover with foil. Bake 30 minutes. Remove foil, continue to bake approximately 10 minutes to brown.

WILD STUFFED PEPPERS

1   pound lean ground buffalo
2   cups cooked wild rice
1   medium onion, chopped
1/2   cup dried fruit bits or raisins
1   cup fat free Swiss cheese, shredded
1   teaspoon salt
1   teaspoon pepper
1   teaspoon cinnamon
6   green peppers

Preheat oven to 350 degrees. Cut green peppers in half and remove stems and seeds. Combine the rest of the ingredients. Lightly stuff the green pepper halves with the wild rice mixture. Place in baking dish and loosely cover with foil. Bake 30 minutes. Uncover, bake 10 minutes or until pepper is tender. 6 servings.

WILD RICE TURKEY OSCAR

1	lb. turkey breast tenderloins
6	ounces imitation crab meat
4	oz. fat free cheese, shredded
1	tablespoon lemon juice
1	teaspoon Dijon mustard
4	cups water
1 1/2	cups <u>uncooked</u> wild rice
1	tablespoon instant chicken bouillon
1	tablespoon chopped fresh tarragon or 1 tsp. dried
1/2	cup raisins
1	15 oz. can asparagus spears
	vegetable spray
	white wine sauce from page 203

Preheat oven to 325 degrees. Spray 9" x 13" pan with vegetable spray. With a sharp knife make a pocket in the long side of tenderlion pieces; cut to within 1/2" of each end. In a medium bowl combine crab, cheese, lemon juice and mustard. Stuff about 1/3 of crab filling in each pocket. Pin together with toothpicks. Place in prepared pan. Spoon remaining filling over top of stuffed tenderlins. Cover with foil and bake about 45 minutes. Uncover; bake 15-20 min. until turkey is done.

Meanwhile, in large saucepan bring water to a boil. Add wild rice, bouillon and tarragon. Cover and simmer 45 minutes, or until rice is tender and grains are starting to puff open. Drain. Stir in raisins. Heat asparagus spears

Spoon wild rice onto large serving platter. Slice each turkey tenderloin into 6 slices. Arrange slices over wild rice. Top with wine sauce and asparagus spears; garnigh with fresh tarragon, if desired. 6 servings.

WILD RICE BREAKFAST BREAD

1/4   cup brown sugar
4   egg whites
1   teaspoon vanilla
1 1/2   cups well-cooked wild rice
1/2   cup chopped raisins
3/4   cup whole wheat flour
3/4   cup white flour
1   teaspoon baking powder
1   teaspoon salt
2   teaspoons cinnamon
3/4   cup skimmed milk
        vegetable spray

Preheat oven to 325 degrees. Add eggs and sugar and beat until fluffy. Add vanilla. Stir in wild rice and raisins. Mix dry ingredients together; add alternately with the milk; stir just until dry ingredients are moistened. Pour mixture into an 8" x 4" veggie sprayed loaf pan. Bake 55-60 minutes. Serve with raspberry jam.

* Note: When combining sugar and wild rice, it is essential to cook wild rice very well. Wild rice has a unique property. Combining with sugar causes the wild rice to revert to a hard kernel. "Over" cooking the wild rice prior to combining with sugar solves this problem.

NORTHWOODS BUTTERMILK CAKE

2   cups well-cooked wild rice
1   cup whole wheat flour
2   cups all-purpose flour
2   teaspoons baking soda
1/2   teaspoon salt
1/2   teaspoon nutmeg

1	cup prunes or dates, pureed in 1/2 cup water
1	cup packed brown sugar
1	teaspoon vanilla
8	egg whites
1/2	cup raisins
1/3	cup applesauce
1	cup buttermilk
	vegetable spray

Preheat oven to 350 degrees. Veggie spray and lightly flour 9" x 13" pan. In medium bowl stir together flours, baking soda, salt, and nutmeg.

In another bowl add brown sugar and vanilla; add eggs, 1 at a time, beating 1 minute after each (batter will look curdled). Add raisins and applesauce blending well after each. Add dry ingredients and buttermilk alternately to mixture, blending well. Stir in wild rice. Turn into prepared pan. Bake 45-50 minutes or till done. Do not overbake. Cool. Frost with a favorite frosting or top each serving with whipped cream from page 317. 12 large servings.

NORTH COUNTRY WILD RICE PANCAKES

1	cup Egg Beaters® egg substitutes
1 1/4	cups buttermilk
1/2	teaspoon baking soda
1 1/4	cups all-purpose flour
1	teaspoon baking powder
1/2	teaspoon salt
1	teaspoon sugar
1	cup cooked wild rice
	vegetable spray

In a large bowl, whisk together the eggs, buttermilk and baking soda. Mix flour, baking powder, salt and sugar and add to the egg mixture. Whisk in the willd rice. Cook pancakes on hot veggie sprayed griddle until golden on both sides. Serve with maple syrup.

NOTE: For thicker pancakes, use only 1/2 cup egg substitute.

WILD RICE FANCY

1 1/2   cups cooked wild rice
1/2   cup packed brown sugar
1/2   cup dates, chopped
1/2   cup marashino cherries, halved
        whipped cream

Combine wild rice, brown sugar, dates and cherries. Chill. Serve with whipped cream from page 317.

NOTE: Prepare in advance to let flavors blend. 4 to 6 servings.

Variation: also good served with milk as a cold cereal.

MEXICALI WILD RICE CASSEROLE   3 +

This quick-to-make casserole features the popular ingredients of Mexican foods with wild rice in a meatless, main dish entree. Vegetarians, as well as those who are trying to eat foods which are low in cholesterol, will like this recipe!

2   cups cooked wild rice
1   (about 17 oz) can whole kernel corn, drained

1   (about 4 oz) can chopped or diced green
        chiles, drained
2   cups (16 oz) chunky, mild salsa sauce
        (use medium for hotter flavor)
1   cup grated cheese (fat free)
        Corn or tortilla chips from page 106 (nachos).

Combine the cooked wild rice with the corn and chilies and spread in a lightly oiled 7" x 11" casserole. Spread the salsa sauce over this and sprinkle with the cheese. Cover and heat at 350 degrees about 30 minutes. Serve with a basket of baked corn or tortilla chips. Serves 4 as a main dish casserole.

To serve individual servings, heat the casserole ingredients without the cheese and spoon over corn or tortilla chips on individual plates; sprinkle cheese on top and, if desired, heat eigher under a broiler or in a microwave to melt cheese.

LEMON WILD RICE CONSOMME

This simple beef consomme with the light lemony taste and the filling, nutritious grains of wild rice could be just for you!

4   cups clear beef broth
4   tsps. fresh lemon juice
1   cup shredded Boston of leaf lettuce
2   cups cooked wild rice
8-12   slivers of lemon peel or 4 thin lemon slices
        (2 or 3 slivers or 1 slice per serving)

Heat beef broth and lemon juice until very hot or just to a boil, but do not allow to boil for any amount of time. Place 1/4 cup shredded lettuce and 1/2 cup wild rice in each of 4 soup cups or bowls. Divide slivers of lemon peel and/or lemon slices in each bowl. Dividing evenly, pour hot beef liquid over other soup ingredients and serve immediately. Serves 4.

NOTE: soup can be served cold or at room temperature, but beef broth and lemon juice should be heated together and allowed to cool to room temperature. If serving soup this way, do not combine lettuce and bro th until broth is cooled to room temperature.

WILD RICE MEDITERRANEAN WITH TUNA

Fresh herbs, garlic, onion and fresh fish are some of the earthy flavors of Provence, a part of southern France that touches the Mediterrean Sea. In this recipe, these country and seaside flavors are combined with one of the most unique American foods, wild rice. Complement this main dish with fresh sliced tomatoes, and good French bread.

2	cups cooked wild rice
1	cup unpeeled zucchini, cut into 1/4 inch slices
1/2	cup coarsely chopped red onion
1/4	cup chicken broth (defatted)
4	garlic cloves, pressed or very finely chopped
1/2	tsp. mixed dried herbs, such as thyme, parsley, summer savory or oregano (or 1/2 cup mixed fresh summer herbs, bruised and very finely chopped)
2	fresh grilled or broiled tuna steaks, or 1 (6 1/2 oz, packed in water) can chunk tuna, drained.

Prepare wild rice, zucchini and red onion. Heat chicken broth with the garlic, salt and herbs, pressing with the back of a wooden spoon

189

to extract flavors. Add zucchini and onion and saute about 1 minute, turning gently once. Add cooked wild rice and saute until heated through. Do not overcook vegetables. Serve hot as a side dish with fresh tuna steaks, using fresh parsley and herbs to garnish. Serves 2.

If fresh tuna is not available, drain the can of tuna and reserve the nicest whole chunks. Divide the remaining pieces of tuna on two individual serving plates or a platter and top with hot wild rice and zucchini mixture. Arrange the reserved chunks of tuna on top and garnish with fresh parsley and/or herbs. Serves 2.

WILD RICE AND SPINACH SALAD

With a hearty bread and fruit for dessert, this main dish salad can be a lunch or dinner entree that is low in fat and high in nutrition. The soy-flavored salad dressing adds an Oriental flavor.

2	cups cooked wild rice, drained well and cooled
2	cups fresh spinach, torn into bite-sized pieces
1/2	cup thinly sliced green onion
1/2	cup crumbled turkey bacon with grease pressed out with a paper towel
2	skinless, defatted chicken breasts, poached and cooled
1/2	cup Italian salad dressing (fat free)
1	tbsp. soy sauce
1/2	tsp. sugar

Prepare the wild rice, spinach, green onion and bacon. Remove meat from chicken breasts in large chunks or "shreds". Combine salad dressing, soy sauce and sugar, stirring to dissolve sugar. If doing salad preparations ahead of time, package and refrigerate each ingredient and dressing separately. When ready to serve, toss all ingredients in a serving bowl adding the dressing during the final tossing. Serves 4.

NOTE: to make a "wilted" salad, heat the dressing before tossing with the ingredients.

WILD RICE AND CARROT MUFFINS

When cooking wild rice, cook some extra to try these carrot and wild rice muffins. With carrots, whole wheat flour and wild rice, these muffins can be a health addition to any mealtime or snack occasion. For sweeter muffins, frost cooled muffins with sweetened cream cheese frosting. (See page 315)

1	cup cooked wild rice
1	cup grated carrots
3/4	cup all-purpose flour
3/4	cup whole wheat flour
2	tsp. baking powder
1/2	tsp. salt
1	tsp. cinnamon
1/2	tsp. nutmeg
1/2	cup brown sugar
2	egg whites, lightly beaten
3/4	cup milk, skimmed
1/2	cup raisins pureed in 1/4 cup water
	veggie spray

For topping:
1	tbsp. sugar
1/4	tsp. cinnamon

Preheat oven to 400 degrees F. Prepare wild rice and carrots and set aside. Combine flours, baking powder, salt, cinnamon, nutmeg and brown sugar together in a mixing bowl, stirring to blend. Add the cooked wild rice to the dry ingredients and toss to coat wild rice.

In another bowl, combine the egg whites with the milk and raisins, add the grated carrots, then stir these wet ingredients into the dry ingredients, mixing just enough to blend well. Do not overmix. Divide batter evenly between 12 veggie sprayed and floured (or paper muffin cup-lined) 2 1/2 inch muffin cups. Mix 1 tbsp. sugar with 1/4 tsp. cinnamon for topping and sprinkle this over muffin batter. Bake at 400 degrees 20 to 25 minutes. Remove muffins from pans and cool on wire racks. Makes 12 muffins.

3. PASTA

Pasta is generally flour, water and some nutrient enriching additives. Never use egg noodles or pasta exceeding 1 gram per 2 oz. (dry weight) portion. Observe the 1 gram per 2 oz. portion and anything goes.

In preparing your pasta never use oil or fat in the cooking process otherwise follow manufacturers directions.

AMERICAN CLASSIC SPAGHETTI

1   Can (27 1/4 oz) Hunt's® Chunky Style
     Spaghetti Sauce
1/2 Cup onions, chopped
1/2 Cup bell pepper, diced
1   Cup fresh whole mushrooms,
     small to medium size
     Pasta, your choice

In sauce pan simmer spaghetti sauce, onions and peppers for 5 minutes. Add mushrooms and simmer for 15 minutes. Spoon onto pasta and serve.

MACARONI & CHEESE

2   Cups dry elbow macaroni
1   Batch cheese sauce page 202
4   Slices fat free cheese

Preheat oven to 375 degrees. Prepare dry macaroni as per package instructions. Remove from stove and drain. Add cheese sauce and put mixture into a 2 quart casserole dish. Cover top with fat free cheese and bake uncovered until top is slightly browned and sauce is bubbling, about 25 minutes.

SEAFOOD MEDLEY WITH FETTUCINI

    Cooked Fettucini for 4
1   Can chicken broth, defatted
1   Cup mixed seafood, cooked
1   Tablespoon parsley, minced
1/4   Cup green onion tops, chopped
1   Tablespoon flour
1/4   Cup crab meat or crab blend
1/2   Cup water
1   Tablespoon dry powdered milk, nonfat
    Salt & white pepper to taste

In blender add 1/2 cup water and crab meat and reduce to puree. Pour into a medium sauce pan, add parsley, onion and powdered non fat milk. Simmer on medium heat for 3 minutes. In bowl mix flour and 1/2 can chicken broth.

Add to sauce pan and simmer gently for 4
minutes. Stir to keep from burning. Remove
from heat and add mixed seafood. Serve on
fettucini.

MACARONI SALAD

2	Cups uncooked elbow macaroni
1	Tablespoon Thousand Island Dressing, fat free
1	Tablespoon pickle relish
1	Tablespoon mayonnaise, fat free
2	Boiled eggs, chopped, discard yolks
	Garnish with sweet pickle slices or
	pickled green tomato slices

Cook macaroni, wash with cold water mix in
the dressing, relish, mayonnaise and eggs.
Garnish top of dish with sweet pickle or pickled
tomato slices.

SMOKED TURKEY FETTUCINI

	Fettucini cooked for 4
1	Cup skimmed milk
1	Can chicken broth, defatted
3	Slices fat free cheese
2	Cups Hickory Smoked skinned turkey breast, cubed
1	Cup whole mushrooms, small to medium size
2	Tablespoons flour
	Salt & white pepper to taste
	Parsley sprigs

In medium sauce pan on medium heat add
milk, 1/2 can chicken broth and turkey. Simmer
for 5 minutes. Add mushrooms and simmer for
5 minutes. Mix thoroughly, flour and 1/2 can
chicken broth, add to sauce pan along with the

cheese. Simmer for 3 minutes. Season to taste and serve on top of fettucini. Garnish with parsley.

TOMATO & CHEESE FETTUCINI

	Cooked fettucini
	Cheese sauce page 202
1/2	Cup green onion tops, chopped
1	Cup fresh tomatoes, bite size pieces
	Salt & pepper to taste

In medium sauce pan on medium heat combine cheese sauce, onion & tomato. Heat to simmer, remove from heat. Season to taste and serve on top of fettucini.

PASTA FIESTA

8	oz. dry multi colored spiral pasta
1	Cup whole mushrooms cooked & marinated
2	Tomatoes, ripe and cut into bite size pieces
1/2	Onion, sliced (sweet onion is best)
1/2	Bell Pepper, bite size pieces
1	Tablespoon red wine vinegar or your favorite non fat dressing
1	Fresh jalapeno pepper, seeded & sliced
1	Teaspoon dry basil

Cook pasta, wash and chill. Boil mushrooms for 5 minutes remove and place in your favorite marinade sauce overnight. If you don't have a favorite, try balsamic vinegar, sliced onion rings and baby beets. Use the beet colored onion rings for your salad. Next day drain mushrooms and combine all ingredients. Toss and serve.

4. DRIED BEANS (LEGUMES)

Beans have been and, continue to be an absolute staple in many parts of the world. When coupled with rice or corn it is the protein source of choice for many peoples. In the orient, the soy bean is almost never eaten as a bean but is consumed as soy sauce, tofu, and many other variations. In our Southwest the pinto bean is preferred; in the Southeast the black-eyed pea; in Boston the navy bean, and if you see a lot of black beans you are probably in South America or the Caribbean.

PREPARATION

Choose the bean you are most comfortable with. Clean and wash. Soak beans overnight and do not discard the soaking water but add to it so as to cover the beans. Gently simmer the beans until tender. Keep the beans adequately covered with water while cooking. Season with flavors you desire. Nonfat bacon flavor works well, onions, peppers (all kinds) tomatoes, salt and molasses continue to be used as traditional seasonings for different beans.

SOUTHWESTERN PINTO BEANS
yields 4 cups *Excellent + easy*

1	Cup dried pinto beans
1/2	Medium onion, diced
1/2	Cup salsa, thick and chunky
1	Fresh jalapeno pepper, sliced (optional)
	Salt to taste

Soak beans overnight. Mix ingredients together and simmer until tender.

MEXICAN PINTO BEANS Excellent
Makes 3 or 4 servings

1   Cup pinto beans, cleaned & washed
2 1/2 Cups hot water
1/2   Teaspoon salt
1/2   Cup onions, diced
1   Teaspoon garlic, minced
1/8   Teaspoon black pepper
1   Tomato, chopped
1/4   Cup green chiles, chopped
1   Teaspoon bacon flavoring

Soak beans overnight, covered with water in a slow electric cooker.

Next morning add all ingredients to pot and set cooker to cook all day.

Serve with warm corn tortillas, rice and green salad.

NEW ORLEANS RED
BEANS AND RICE

2   Cups red kidney beans, cleaned &
       soaked overnight
1/4   Pound lean ham, diced pork or turkey ham
1/2   Tablespoon Molly McButter® Bacon
       flavor sprinkles
1   Tablespoon flour
1   Medium onion chopped
1   Small carrot sliced
6   Cups chicken stock or
       6 cups water with 3 bouillon cubes
1   Bay leaf
1/8   Teaspoon thyme
1/8   Teaspoon sage
1   Teaspoon parsley
1   Stalk celery chopped

197

Salt, pepper and cayenne pepper to taste

In dutch oven brown flour, add onions brown also for 2 or 3 minutes. Add other ingredients and simmer until beans are tender and juice is thick and dark. Correct seasoning and serve over rice.

BOSTON BAKED BEANS
Makes 3 or 4 servings

1	Cup small white beans, cleaned and washed
2 1/2	Cups hot water
1/2	Teaspoon salt
1/2	Cup diced onions
1	Teaspoon minced garlic
1	Tablespoon dark molasses
1	Tablespoon Dijon-style prepared mustard
1/4	Teaspoon thyme
1	Bay leaf
1/2	Teaspoon ginger, powdered
1/8	Teaspoon black pepper
1/2	Teaspoon bacon flavor

Soak beans at least 4 hours then place all ingredients in electric slow cooker set to low or in oven set to 275 degrees F. Cook overnight or 12-14 hours.

Serve with cole slaw, page 113 and fresh bread.

NAVY BEANS & ONIONS
yields 4 cups

1	Cup dried navy beans, washed & soaked
1	Medium onion, chopped
	Salt & black pepper to taste

Soak beans overnight, add onion. Salt and black pepper. Simmer until done. Balance seasonings.

CHILI BEANS

2	Cups dried pinto beans, washed & soaked
1	Medium onion, chopped
2	Tablespoons chili powder
1	Cup salsa, thick & chunky
1	Tablespoon garlic, minced
1	Cup tomatoes, diced
*1/4	Cup Textured Vegetable Protein (TVP®)
1/8	Teaspoon cayenne pepper
	Salt & pepper to taste

Soak beans overnight. Combine ingredients and simmer until tender and water just covers the beans.

*NOTE: Textured Vegetable Protein (TVP®) Takes on the appearance of ground meat, and can be purchased at most health food and specialty stores or by calling 1-800-8-FLAVOR.

BACHELORS
(REALLY Quick) MEXICAN BEANS & RICE
Main Course for Two

1. One 15 oz. can pinto beans
2. 1/2 bean can your favorite Mexican salsa or taco sauce
3. 1 Tablespoon onion soup mix
4. 1/4 bean can of water
5. 1 bean can instant rice
6. 1/2 cup chopped sweet onions
7. 1/2 cup chopped tomatoes

8. Jalapeno pepper slices

Mix first four ingredients in 2 quart or bigger sauce pan and bring to a careful boil. (don't burn the beans). When mixture boils add: 5. One bean can full of minute rice. Remove from burner and let sit for five minutes.
Then add: 6. 1/2 Cup of chopped sweet onions. 7. 1/2 Cup of chopped fresh tomatoes Garnish with jalapeno peppers and serve with steamed or baked corn tortillas.

HOT DOG CHILI

1	Can chile beans
1/2	Medium onions, chopped
1/2	Cup chicken broth, defatted
1/4	Cup thick salsa
	Hormel® Light & Lean® frankfurters

Simmer onion in chicken broth until tender. Add beans, salsa and frankfurters cut into bite sizes. Heat but don't burn. Goes great in a hot dog bun topped with fat free cheese.

VI. SAUCES

In France they say that the sauce is everything. Well, maybe not "everything" but a good sauce can turn an ordinary dish into an elegant dish. Sauces can be part of the heart and soul of good food. Sliced cold breast of turkey when served on a bed of Purple Kale and topped with cranberry wine sauce transcends the ordinary.

To a midwesterner it might be called "cream gravy", in France they would call it Bechamel sauce; add curry powder and it becomes a cream curry sauce; whatever the name the sauce is the game.

BUTTER SAUCE

1	Envelope Butter Buds® Butter Flavored Granules
1/2	Cup water
1	Teaspoon corn starch

Heat in sauce pan or microwave until just boiling. Remove from heat and stir. Will keep covered for 3 days in refrigerator.

Brush on corn-on-the-cob, toast, bread or vegetables.

For garlic butter sauce add 1 teaspoon minced garlic.

WHITE SAUCE OR BECHAMEL SAUCE I
(CREAM GRAVY)

2	Tablespoons flour
1 1/2	Cup non fat milk
1	Teaspoon dry Butter Buds® Butter Flavor Granules

Salt & white pepper to taste

Mix ingredients in blender or whisk in a bowl until mixture is thoroughly blended. Simmer for 5 minutes over low heat.

- **Curry Sauce** add 1 teaspoon curry powder.

- **Cheese Sauce** - while sauce is hot, stir in 4 slices of fat free cheese and allow to melt.

- **Egg Sauce** - Add the chopped whites from 2 hard boiled eggs.

WHITE SAUCE (BECHAMEL) II

2   Teaspoons imitation butter flavor
2   Tablespoons flour
1   Can evaporated skim milk
      Salt & pepper to taste

Combine ingredients in sauce pan and whisk briskly in order to thoroughly mix. Heat over medium heat, stirring all the time until sauce is thick and smooth. Simmer for 2 or 3 minutes and remove from heat.

Hot Mustard Sauce. Stir in 2 teaspoons of hot Chinese mustard powder.

Tame Mustard Sauce. Stir in 2 tablespoons mustard of your choice.

Cheese Sauce. While sauce is hot, stir in 2 slices of fat free cheese and allow to melt.

Egg Sauce. Add the chopped whites from 2 hard boiled eggs.

Parsley Sauce. Add 1/2 cup finely chopped parsley after sauce is done.

Caper Sauce. Add capers to suit your taste to the finished sauce.

White Wine Sauce. When cooking sauce, add 1/4 cup white wine.

Champagne Sauce. Saute one medium onion (chopped fine) and 1/2 bell pepper in 1/4 cup champagne for 10 minutes. Add white sauce. Strain if desired.

Tomato-Basil Cream Sauce. Add 1/2 cup chopped Tomato pulp from canned Italian plum tomatoes and 1 tablespoon fresh basil (or 1 teaspoon dried basil) to white sauce.

Tarragon Sauce. Add 2 teaspoons dried tarragon and 1 tablespoon white wine. Serve over broiled breast of chicken.

White Clam Sauce. Add cooked, chopped clams to taste. Add reduced clam broth if desired.

BROWN SAUCE

1	Teaspoon flour
4	Ounces sliced ham (diced)
1	Medium onion, diced
1	Carrot, thinly sliced
2	Cups beef broth
1	Teaspoon imitation butter flavor
1/2	Bay leaf
1/8	Teaspoon dried thyme
1/4	Cup tomato sauce

1/4   Cup red wine
        Salt & pepper to taste

In cast iron skillet brown flour and ham over medium heat. Add onions, carrots and a little beef broth and cook until onions are brown. Add the rest of the beef broth, bay leaf, butter flavor, thyme and simmer for 1 hour. Add tomato sauce, wine and simmer for another 1/2 hour. Salt & pepper to taste and strain through a sieve. If sauce isn't thick enough continue to simmer until it is.

MADEIRA BROWN SAUCE

Add Madeira to Brown Sauce.

MUSHROOM BROWN SAUCE

Saute desired amount and type of sliced mushrooms in a little water. Boil off water and add to Madeira Brown Sauce.

SAUCE DIABLO

To one cup Brown Sauce, add 1 teaspoon hot Chinese mustard powder, 1 teaspoon tabasco, 1/4 teaspoon black pepper and 1 teaspoon fresh lemon juice. Simmer for a few minutes to mix flavors.

BORDELAISE SAUCE

Reduce 1 cup of red wine to 1/2 cup, add six chopped green onions and 1 cup of brown sauce. *Goes great on a Buffalo steak!*

LEMON BUTTER SAUCE

	Grated rind of 1/2 lemon
2	Tablespoons fresh lemon juice
1/4	Cup Chicken Broth
1/2	Cup Butter Buds® Butter flavor liquid mixture
1	Teaspoon corn starch
1	Teaspoon chopped herbs such as parsley, dill or chives

Bring lemon rind, juice and chicken broth to a boil and simmer until reduced to about 3 tablespoons of liquid. Combine Butter Buds® liquid and corn starch thoroughly then add to juice and simmer for a minute or so. Add herbs and serve over fish.

ONION BUTTER SAUCE

1	Cup water
1/2	Envelope onion soup mix
1	Envelope (1/2 oz.) Butter Buds® Butter flavored granules
2	Teaspoons corn starch

Mix and simmer in sauce pan for 5 minutes. Store covered in refrigerator. May be used as topping for toasted french bread, on baked or mashed potatoes or on pasta.

HORSERADISH SAUCE

1	Cup light sour cream
1/4	Cup horseradish

Mix and chill
Great with roast beef.

FLUFFY HORSERADISH SAUCE

Goes great with a medium rare prime rib of buffalo.

1/2	Cup sour cream from page 321
1/3	Cup nonfat milk powder
4	Tablespoons prepared horseradish
1/4	Teaspoon salt
	Pepper to taste

Whip sour cream and milk powder until stiff; fold in horseradish, salt and pepper.

SOUR CREAM MUSTARD SAUCE

1	Cup light sour cream
1	Teaspoon prepared mustard
2	Tablespoons green onion tops, minced or
1	Tablespoon regular onion
	Salt & pepper to taste

Mix, chill and serve.

Goes well with fish, fowl or veggies.

TARTAR SAUCE

1	Cup fat free mayonnaise
2	Tablespoon minced onion
1/2	Cup dill pickle, finely minced
1	Teaspoon capers, minced
1/8	Teaspoon cayenne pepper

Mix and chill
Great with fish.

CUCUMBER CREAM SAUCE

1   Cup light sour cream
1/4   Cup cucumber
1/8   Cup water
1   Tablespoon vinegar
      Salt to taste

In blender, puree cucumber and water. Remove to bowl and add sour cream, vinegar and salt to taste.

HEAVY CREAM DESSERT SAUCE

Simple Pleasure® Light Frozen Vanilla Dairy Dessert made with the all natural fat substitute Simplesse®

Allow desired amount to thaw in refrigerator or hurry along in the microwave.

Serve on desserts such as shortcakes, cake, berries or parfaits.

MUSHROOM SAUCE

     White sauce page 202
1   Cup mushrooms, sliced
1   Teaspoon chicken bouillon powder
1/4   Cup water

Simmer mushrooms, water and bouillon until water is almost boiled away. Add to white sauce and serve.

HOLLANDAISE SAUCE

1/2	Cup Egg Beaters® egg substitute
2	Tablespoons lemon juice
3	Tablespoons Butter Buds® Butter flavor granules
3/4	Cup evaporated skim milk
2	Teaspoons cornstarch
1	Tablespoon parsley
	Salt & cayenne pepper to taste

In mixing bowl mix thoroughly with whisk or mixer. Pour into sauce pan and bring to simmer over medium heat stirring continuously with whisk.

SAUSAGE GRAVY

Sausage patties page 136.
White sauce page 202

In skillet crumble sausage patties and brown. Add white sauce. Stir, remove from heat and let sit for 5 minutes. If thinner gravy is desired, add more skim milk. Serve over hot biscuits, page 266.

COLE SLAW DRESSING

1/2	Cup fat free mayonnaise
1	Tablespoon cider vinegar
1	Tablespoon sugar
1	Teaspoon non fat dry milk solids
1	Teaspoon Butter Buds® Butter flavor granules

CRANBERRY-WINE SAUCE

1/8   Cup burgundy wine
1   16 oz. Can cranberry sauce
2   Tablespoons light brown sugar
1   Tablespoon prepared mustard
1/8   Teaspoon onion salt

Combine all ingredients and simmer for 3 minutes. Serve with sliced breast of turkey or chicken. May be served chilled.

BASIC GRAVY

1   cup liquid
1 1/4   tablespoon flour
          seasonings

Combine in sauce pan or skillet beef or chicken broth with flour and mix thoroughly. Heat to boil and simmer for 3 or 4 minutes. Season to taste. For thicker gravy use more flour.

VII. SANDWICHES, TACOS, BURRITOS, AND PIZZA

Sandwiches are the mainstay of our society. Both standard sandwiches and latin varieties make our country functional. Without sandwiches, many people would become disoriented, confused, and unable to perform routine tasks. Some would probably starve. For these reasons, we include this life-saving section.

SANDWICHES

Always purchase fat-free bread! There are many brands and styles of fat-free bread to choose from, of course homemade fat-free bread provides something special to any sandwich.

HOT TURKEY TOMATO MELT

Breast of turkey, sliced
Tomato
Fat-free cheese
English muffins

Pile turkey on to muffin, add tomato, top with cheese, and broil until cheese melts. Serve hot.

BACON CHEESE BURGER
For Two

2   defatted beef patties, buffalo, or venison
4   strips turkey bacon
2   slices fat-free cheese
    Salt and pepper

Cook bacon crisp and place on paper towel. Press to remove fat. In skillet, place small amount of water and beef patties; simmer to heat. Season to taste. Place a slice of cheese on each patty, cover and allow to just melt. Remove from skillet to bun and top dress with two strips of bacon for each patty.

MUSHROOM CHEESEBURGER

2   cooked defatted beef patties
2   cups sliced fresh mushrooms
1   teaspoon beef bouillon powder
2   slices fat-free cheese
           Salt and pepper

In heavy skillet, place small amount of water and add mushrooms. Sprinkle with beef bullion. Place beef patties on top of mushrooms and simmer until mushrooms are done. Arrange mushrooms to tops of patties, season to taste and cover with cheese slices. Cover skillet in order to melt cheese. Serve on homemade bread slices or buns.

PHILLY BEEF AND CHEESE

1/4   pound defatted roast beef
1/2   cup defatted beef broth
2   slices of large onion
1/2   sliced bell pepper
1/2   cup fat-free mozzarella cheese
           Salt and pepper

Slice roast beef wafer thin. In heavy skillet, add broth, beef, onions, and peppers and simmer five minutes or until peppers are "as you like them". Add cheese and mix thoroughly. Spoon on to toasted buns. Makes 2 sandwiches.

BAR-B-QUE BEEF SANDWICH

2   cups shredded beef page 124
1/2   cup defatted beef broth
1   cup your favorite bar-b-que sauce

In sauce pan, heat beef and beef broth. Add bar-b-que sauce and lower heat to just warm. Allow to warm for 5 to 10 minutes. Spoon mixture onto buns and serve.

HOT BEEF SANDWICH

Roast beef and gravy from page 123 , sliced very thin
Mashed potatoes page 169

Heat and assemble "open-face" style

SLOPPY JOES

1   packet of Midland Harvest Burger Mix®
      (to obtain Midland Harvest Burger Mix®,
      see chapter 9)
1   can or jar sloppy joe sauce.

Reconstitute burger mix and brown in skillet. Add sauce and serve.

CHILI DOGS

Hot dogs, Hormel® Light & Lean® Frankfurters
Chili beans from can or chili from page 199
Hot dog buns

Place beans and hot dogs in sauce pan and heat. Place hot dog in bun and top with chili.

For slaw dogs substitute cole slaw
for chili.

HOT DOGS AND SAUERKRAUT

Hormel® Light & Lean® hot dogs
Canned sauerkraut
Hot dog buns
Mustard

In large skillet, heat sauerkraut and hot dogs.
Place a plate of hot dog buns in the center of
skillet, cover and allow buns to warm. Serve
with mustard.

HOT TURKEY SANDWICH

Turkey and gravy from page 123
Mashed potatoes from page 169
Cranberry sauce

Heat and assemble "open-face" style.

BACON, LETTUCE, AND TOMATO (BLT)

Turkey bacon
Lettuce
Tomato
Fat-free mayonnaise

Fry bacon crisp and remove all visible grease
from bacon with paper towels. Assemble
sandwich.

FISH SANDWICH

Fish fillet, baked with Shake N' Bake®
Seasoning and Coating Original Recipe for fish

Fat-free cheese
Tartar Sauce, page206

Top fish with cheese, spread on tarter sauce.

FRIED HAM AND CHEESE

Turkey ham slices
Dill pickle slices
Lettuce
Tomato
Fat-free mayonnaise

Fry ham and press with paper towel to remove fat. Assemble sandwich.

FRIED HAM AND EGG

Sliced turkey ham
Egg Beaters® egg substitutes
Lettuce
Tomato
Pickle
Fat-free mayonnaise

Fry ham and press with paper towel to remove fat. Fry egg and assemble.

TACOS

Do not purchase prepared taco shells unless they are clearly marked "fat free". Purchase corn tortillas and form and bake your own. If simplicity is desired, lay tortillas flat on cookie sheet and bake for 20 minutes at 325 degrees. These will make open face tacos or tostadas.

BEAN TACOS

Refried beans, page 225
Baked tortillas
Shredded lettuce
Chopped tomatoes
Chopped onions
Shredded fat-free mozzarella cheese

Spread hot refried beans on tortilla. Top with other ingredients.

NOTE: For chicken or turkey tacos, use meat from page 123 or low-fat deli slices. For meat tacos, use meat from page 124 or 1 gram per slice deli beef luncheon meat.

SOFT TACOS

Use fat-free flour tortillas or quick flour tortillas page 266 , assemble as for corn tortilla tacos and fold in half.

BURRITOS

Traditionally in Mexico and parts of the Southwest, the burrito, for lunch, is nothing more than unleavened   bread wrapped around last night's leftovers. It might be filled with beans, rice, corn, liver, meat, poultry, tripe, cheese, fish, or combinations of leftovers. Potatoes are often cooked, diced, and mixed with eggs and chilies and used as a filling for a burrito. When wrapped in aluminum foil and taken to work in the lunch bucket, a construction worker can have a hot lunch by placing the wrapped burrito on top of a hot engine. Americanized versions show up as deep fried or baked with various toppings. So, let your imagination go to work and just exclude any fatty ingredients.

BEAN BURRITO WITH CHILES AND CHEESE

Fat-free flour tortillas or from page 266
Refried beans from page 225
Fat-free cheese
Salsa or taco sauce
Green chilies

Spread beans on tortilla, add cheese, chilies, and salsa. Roll up and wrap in aluminum foil. Place in warm oven and allow cheese to melt. May be prepared well in advance. Any extra can go to work the next day in the lunch box.

SCRAMBLED EGG AND POTATO BURRITO

Egg Beaters® egg substitute
Fat-free flour tortilla or from page 266
Diced onions
Diced potatoes
Beef broth
Green chilies
Salsa
Salt and pepper to taste

Simmer onions, potatoes, green chilies, and beef broth until potatoes are done and beef broth is completely reduced. Scramble Egg Beaters® and assemble burrito. Wrap in aluminum foil if desired.

GREEN PEON BURRITO

       Fat-free frozen or fresh hash-brown potatoes
1   4 oz can chopped green chiles
       Thick salsa or taco sauce
       Salt and pepper to taste
       Flour tortillas

In large veggie-sprayed skillet, place desired amount of potatoes and brown over medium heat. When browned, add green chiles and stir while warming chiles. Remove from heat and place tortillas on top of mixture in order to warm. Cover skillet and allow to sit for a few minutes. Place skillet in the center of dining table and let people make their own burritos. Serve with salsa or taco sauce.

RED CHILE VEGGIE-BURGER BURRITO

1/2   lb. Midland Harvest Burger®
       Mix, reconstituted
1/2   medium sliced onion
1/4   cup thick salsa or taco sauce
2   slices fat-free cheese
4   teaspoons enchilada sauce mix
       Flour tortillas

On medium heat, veggie spray a cast-iron skillet and spoon veggie burger into center of skillet. Place onion slices around outer edges. sprinkle enchilada sauce mix onto top of burger mix. Brown burger, mix and turn over adding salsa or taco sauce. Cover and allow to steam for a few minutes. Add more onions into the mixture if desired and allow to cook through. Break cheese into pieces and add to mixture so it doesn't stick to the tortillas and place tortillas on top and cover. Remove from heat and allow time for tortillas to warm.

RED CHILE CHICKEN BURRITOS
For Two

	Hash-brown potatoes for two (fresh or frozen - but fat free)
	Enchilada sauce mix powder
1	small chopped tomato
4	flour tortillas
	Salt and pepper to taste
	Vegetable spray
1	small chopped onion

In large veggie-sprayed cast-iron skillet, spread hash browns over half of skillet. Coat chicken liberally with enchilada sauce mix and place on the other half of skillet and cook over medium heat. Top chicken with tomatoes as you turn chicken. Add onions to skillet when desired, but keep separate. Salt and pepper hash browns. When done, remove from heat and place tortillas on top and cover skillet. Allow to sit while tortillas warm.
Set skillet on dining table and enjoy.

BAKED BURRITO

Fat-free flour tortillas
Filling of your choice (i.e. meat, poultry, beans, etc.)
Chili beans from page 199 or canned

Assemble burritos and place on cookie sheet. Bake in 400-degree oven for 30 minutes or until brown and crispy. Remove and top with chili beans just before serving. Serve with fresh, chopped jalapeno peppers, low-fat sour cream, and shredded lettuce.

CHICKEN OR TURKEY BURRITO

1   cup breast meat, cooked and shredded
1/4 cup chopped onions
1   cup sliced long green chilies
1/4 cup salsa of your choice
6   slices fat-free cheese singles
6   fat-free flour tortillas or from page 266

DOGGIE BURRITOS

6   corn tortillas or flour, your choice
6   frankfurters, Hormel® Light & Lean®
3   slices fat free cheese
1   can chili beans

Preheat oven to 400 degrees F.

Place frank and 1/2 slice cheese in a tortilla; roll up and hold together with a toothpick. Repeat. Place in oven proof pan and top with beans. Bake for 20 minutes. Serve with shredded lettuce.

NOTE: Beans may be replaced with your favorite salsa and topped with additional slices of cheese.

PIZZAS

From the crust up, pizzas are a fine source of eating contentment. Starting with the crust, "store bought" pizza doughs are fine if they do not contain oil, hydrogenated oils, shortening, or lard. Read the ingredient label carefully. If your can't find fat-free dough in your supermarket, then use any fat-free homemade yeast bread recipe. Just form into pizza crust after the first rising.

Fat-free cheese toppings are fine. If you have an absolute craving for pepperoni, then purchase the wafer thin slices and boil the fat out of them for about 30 minutes. Another meat topping might be smoked turkey sausage, sliced wafer thin and boiled for 30 minutes. ADM Midland Harvest Burger® mix also makes a fine topping. The pizza sauce should comply with the 1 gram per serving rule. Hunt's® Chunky Style Spaghetti Sauce with tomato chunks is a fine sauce for pizzas. Molly McButter® Bacon Flavor and Cheese Flavor add a lot of good flavor to any pizza. The basic rule for fat-free pizza is: Buy proper ingredients and use your imagination.

OUR FAVORITE PIZZA

	Patmos brand prepared pizza dough
	Hunt's® Chunky Style Spaghetti Sauce
6	slices ripe tomato
2	cups sliced mushroom
1	cup sliced bell pepper
1	large sweet onion, sliced
	Molly McButter® bacon and cheese flavors to taste

Assemble and bake at 400 degrees for 25 minutes or until edges are brown and crusty.

VIII. VEGETABLES

The cook said to the King. "This bowl of peppers will go well with your leg of venison". Now the King was not knowledgeable of the nature of red and green cayenne peppers, so unknowingly he did partake of the venison and did dip handily into the bowl of peppers. His temples did throb, he perspired profusely, his lips and mouth were afire, his eyes watered and his throat allowed him not to speak.

When the King finally did recover he had the cook's head lopped off. The moral of this story is -- present your vegetables as they are perceived to be. That is, french fried potatoes should be crisp and brown, buttered carrots should be buttery, sauces should be flavorful and creamy, and so on.

To accomplish these ends, learn to use those "flavor tools" at your disposal that are fat free. As an addition to your vegetables, consider the bacon and cheese sprinkles, the cheddar cheeses, Butter Buds® butter flavored granules, Mozzarella cheese, American cheese, dry soup mixes (especially onion and vegetable soup), along with the always available fresh mushrooms and onions.

Don't be afraid to experiment, just don't shock the King.

PEAS AND MUSHROOMS

2	Cups frozen or fresh peas
1	Cup sliced mushrooms
1/4	Cup baby onions or chopped onions
1	Teaspoon Butter Buds® Butter Flavored Granules
1	Teaspoon sugar

1   Tablespoon chopped red bell pepper
1/4   Cup water

Cook peas as directed or until tender and drain. Cook onions, mushrooms and red bell pepper in 1/4 cup water until tender.
Mix all ingredients together, cover and heat through.

CREAMED PEAS

1   Package frozen peas cooked & drained
       White sauce from page 201

Combine, warm and serve.

GREEN KALE & DUMPLINGS

2   Tablespoons beef bouillon granules
4   Teaspoons Molly McButter® Bacon flavor
2   lbs Kale
3   Slices turkey ham cut in strips
1   lb. potatoes, diced in one inch cubes
2   Ears of sweet corn cut into thirds
10   Cups water
       Dumpling batter page 285
       Salt & pepper to taste

Remove stems from kale and in a large dutch oven or kettle bring water to boil, add kale, potatoes, ham, corn, and bacon flavor and simmer for 20 minutes. Spoon in large tablespoons of dumpling batter so as to make about a dozen dumplings. Cover and simmer for an additional 30 minutes or until dumplings are done. Serve greens and broth in bowl topped with dumplings. Serve corn on the side brushed with Butter Sauce page 201.

BROCCOLI-CAULIFLOWER SOUFFLE

1	Cup chopped broccoli
1	Cup chopped cauliflower
1	Teaspoon Butter Buds® Butter Flavored Granules
2	Tablespoons flour
1/2	Teaspoon salt
1/2	Cup non fat milk
6	Slices fat free cheese
1	Cup Egg Beaters® egg substitutes

In salted water, cook broccoli and cauliflower 10 minutes, drain well. Blend milk, Butter Buds®, and flour, cook and stir until bubbly, remove from heat. Add cheese stir until blended then add broccoli and cauliflower. Beat eggs at high speed for 4 minutes, and add to veggies. Spoon into an ungreased 1 quart souffle dish. Bake at 350 degrees for 35 minutes until a knife inserted comes out clean. Serve immediately.

REFRIED BEAN CASSEROLE

Pinto beans
Fat free cheese
Salt & pepper to taste

Mash beans and season. Spoon into casserole dish and cover top with cheese slices. Bake in 350 degree oven until beans are hot and cheese is bubbly.

CORN POPOVERS

1	Cup canned corn, whole kernel drained
1	Popover recipe page 265

Add corn to Popover batter and spoon into veggie sprayed muffin tins. Bake as per Popover recipe.

CANDIED RAISIN-SWEET POTATOES

Sweet potatoes, as desired
Raisins
Brown sugar

Place desired amount of sweet potatoes in casserole dish with raisins, sprinkle liberally with brown sugar and bake at 350 degrees until done.

TOMATO-MUSHROOM QUICHE

4	Strips turkey bacon, cooked crisp & drained of fat
1	Cup fresh ripe tomatoes, chopped
1	Cup fresh mushrooms, sliced
1	Teaspoon Molly McButter® Bacon flavor granules
1	Cup Egg Beaters® egg substitutes
2	Cups evaporated non fat milk
1/2	Teaspoon salt
1/8	Teaspoon nutmeg
	Dash cayenne pepper
1	Cup grated mozzarella cheese (non fat)
4	Slices fat free cheese
2	Pie shells page 278, uncooked

Heat oven to 425 degrees. Place tomatoes, pieces of bacon, and mushrooms into 2 pie shells. Sprinkle with bacon flavor. Heat milk and cheese until cheese melts. Do not burn! Beat eggs for 1 minute then add to milk. Pour over tomatoes and mushrooms and bake for 15 minutes then lower heat to 350 degrees and continue to bake for 30 minutes or until knife inserted in center comes out clean. Serve hot or cold.

NOTE: These quiches are as variable as your imagination. You might try:

> Smoked turkey & mushrooms
> Bacon-spinach
> Crab & red bell pepper
> Tuna-onion
> Ham & fresh green beans
> Asparagus & lobster blend

Just pour the milk, egg & cheese liquid on top of other choice ingredients.

GREEN BEAN CASSEROLE

1	Cheese sauce page 202.
1	Tablespoon beef bouillon granules
1	Teaspoon soy sauce
2	Green onions, chopped
2	9 oz. package frozen green beans cooked & drained

Combine ingredients and spoon into casserole dish. Bake at 350 degrees for 30 minutes.

SNAPPY THREE PEPPER CORN

1	Can whole kernel corn
1/4	Cup green bell peppers, chopped
1	Tablespoon pimento pepper, chopped (or red bell pepper)
3-4	Slices jalapeno pepper
	Salt and pepper to taste

Combine ingredients in sauce pan and simmer for 5 minutes.

CABBAGE & SAUERKRAUT

For ages, cabbage has been the winter green vegetable of choice. The reason being that cabbage keeps well in the root cellar. It also keeps well if you shred it into a barrel and allow it to ferment as in sauerkraut. An eastern european person probably couldn't exist without cabbage. It shows up in many dishes. Almost every day cabbage shows up in soup, stews, slaws, salads, and in sandwiches. How about sauerkraut and sausage, cabbage and pork, sauerkraut and pork and in Poland, sauerkraut, cabbage and pork. The combinations and uses found for cabbage are apparently endless.

I like to keep a bag of shredded cabbage in the refrigerator. It keeps really well and it is easy to grab a handful when making a fast soup or stew. Or throw a couple of handfuls into a skillet, splash on some liquid, add some vinegar and sugar and you have a tangy addition to many meat dinners.

One tip on cabbage you might remember is that it gets stronger in flavor the longer it cooks and some people find this objectionable. When steaming cabbage cook it until it is just tender, maybe just not quite tender.

SWEET CABBAGE & SOUR BEETS

3	Handfuls shredded cabbage
1	Can whole beets
3	Tablespoons vinegar
3	Tablespoons sugar

1   Tablespoon cornstarch mixed with
        1/4 cup water

In skillet boil cabbage, beets, beet juice, vinegar and sugar until cabbage is just tender. Don't over cook! Pour in cornstarch and water mixture and continue heating until liquid thickens.

STEAMED CABBAGE WEDGES

Cabbage wedges
Chicken broth, defatted
Black pepper
Butter Buds® flavor granules
Chopped parsley

Place cabbage in sauce pan with enough broth to steam. Sprinkle with pepper, flavoring and parsley.
Simmer until tender.

TERIYAKI CABBAGE
(for 2)

2   Handsful shredded cabbage
2   Tablespoons teriyaki sauce
1/4   Cup chicken broth
1/2   Cup broccoli florets
1   Handful bean sprouts
        Teriyaki glaze (bought in supermarket)

In hot skillet or wok steam cabbage, broccoli, teriyaki sauce, and chicken broth. Add bean sprouts at the end of the process to just warm good. Remove from heat. Serve over rice topped with teriyaki glaze to taste.

STEAMED SHREDDED CABBAGE

Shredded Cabbage, (desired amount)
Chicken broth to steam
Salt & pepper to taste

In skillet over medium heat add cabbage and broth. Cover and steam until desired doneness is achieved. Salt and pepper after it is cooked.

NOTE: Pre shredded cabbage or cole slaw mix in a plastic bag available at most produce departments works well and saves time.

SPINACH CASSEROLE SUPREME

1/2	Cup Egg Beaters® egg substitute
1	15 oz. Spinach (drained)
1	Cup riccota cheese
4	Slices Fat Free cheese
1	Tablespoon minced garlic
1/8	Teaspoon white pepper
1	Teaspoon chicken bouillon granules
1/4	Cup chopped onions
1/2	Cup chopped fresh tomatoes

Preheat oven to 400 degrees F.
Except for cheese slices, combine ingredients and plae in a 2 quart casserole dish. Top with cheese slices and bake for 35 minutes.

ROASTED GREEN CHILES

Place long green chiles (anaheims) under broiler and broil until brown and puffy. Turn and brown the other side. Remove and cool. Peel skin from peppers and remove seeds. Skin should peel off easily. If not you probably didn't brown them enough.

LEEKS

I call leeks the lonely vegetable because I never see anybody buy them, I didn't buy them because my Mother didn't buy them and I didn't eat them and my friends didn't eat them. Maybe your mother didn't buy them either and you don't. Here's a reason to give them a try.

Leeks have a wonderful onion family flavor that accentuates the flavor of potatoes and sour cream. If that sounds like a peculiar combination of flavors, I ask you to consider your baked potato with sour cream and chives. Leeks are giant chives or chives are midget leeks, I think. Anyhow, when you simmer leeks and potatoes together you end up with a wonderful soup that is about as simple as simple gets. Ladled up fresh from the soup pot, topped with a spoon of sour cream and served with fresh homemade bread, you have true gourmet fare that is elegant and easy.

LEEK AND POTATO SOUP
3 to 4 servings

2	Cups leeks, sliced including some tender green part
2	Cups potatoes, diced
3	Cups water
1/2	Teaspoon salt
1/4	Cup evaporated skim milk, (optional)
	Sour cream

In a heavy sauce pan, bring leeks, potatoes, water and salt to a boil, cover and simmer for 30

minutes. Add milk and remove from heat. Correct seasoning. Serve hot with a spoonful of sour cream on top.
NOTE: For Vichyssoise serve chilled.

SAVORY SPINACH

2	Packages frozen spinach, chopped
1/4	Cup cream cheese from page 322
1	Cup fresh mushrooms, sliced
1	Tablespoon flour
1/2	Cup evaporated skim milk
1/2	Medium onion, diced
1/4	Cup chicken broth
	Salt and pepper to taste

In a large sauce pan gently simmer onions and broth until onions are tender. Add spinach, mushrooms and simmer until tender. combine milk and flour and add to pan. Remove when thickened and add cream cheese cut into small pieces, stir but don't boil. Season to taste and serve.

LEMON BABY CARROTS

2	Cups baby carrots
	Juice from 1/2 lemon
1	Teaspoon Butter Buds® flavor granules
	Water to boil or chicken broth

In a sauce pan add carrots, lemon juice and enough water to cover carrots. Boil until tender, sprinkle with Butter Buds® flavor and serve.

GLAZED CARROTS

Remove carrots from previous recipe to oven proof serving dish add 1/4 cup brown sugar, toss and place under broiler until brown and bubbly.

QUICK CHILI
(no meat)

1/2	Pound Midland Harvest Burger® or
3	Tablespoons TVP®
1/2	Can chicken broth
1	Can chili beans
2	Teaspoons chili powder (or more to taste)
1	Small can tomatoes
	Vegetable spray

In veggie sprayed skillet, brown veggie burger. Add other ingredients and simmer for 5 minutes.

COLE SLAW II
(for 2)

2	Cups shredded cabbage
4	Tablespoons fat free mayonnaise
4	Tablespoons canned evaporated skim milk
3	Teaspoons vinegar
	(red wine vinegar is fine)
1	Packet artificial sweetener or sugar to taste

Combine and refrigerate.

IX. BREAD

A nybody can make bread, but why would anyone want to?

The task of bread making probably originated in our pre-agricultural history, while we were still hunting and gathering. Smooth river stones were used to grind and pulverize gathered seeds, grain, and nuts. The resultant meal was then mixed with water and wild seasonings, placed on a hot rack, and allowed to steam and bake. This cooking process rendered the ingredients more digestible and un-wittingly created stronger bonds among family members. The act of "Breaking Bread" together was, and is, a celebration of man's victory over the elements. To gather, to prepare, and to share. Each family member had an important responsibility in the act of survival, and one of those responsibilities was the making of bread.

Turn-of-the-Century farm life was entirely dependent upon homemade breads. Often times it was Grandma, arising at 4:30 - 5:00 a.m., who slipped deftly into the quiet kitchen to coax the wood cookstove back to life using kindling brought in the night before by one of the young men. Soon the "quick breads" in the form of biscuits, pancakes, griddle cakes, and waffles were mixed and cooking.

As the coffee began to boil, the household sprang to life. The older boys followed Dad to milk the cows. The older girls help the younger children get dressed for school. When those tasks were accomplished, everyone filed into the kitchen to assist in different ways with the preparation of the day's food. The sorghum molasses pot was refilled, a new jar of apple butter was retrieved from the cellar along with a jar of spiced peaches, and everyone sat down to break the night-long fast by partaking of and giving thanks for the daily bread.

After the kitchen was cleaned, it was Mom's turn to shine in the bread-making department. The "sponge" that was prepared the night before was uncovered and, sure enough, the mixture consisting of a yeast starter, flour, molasses, and water had created a large bowl full of a bubbling, aerated, growing mass of yeast and flour. More water was added along with salt, left-over mashed potatoes, and flour. Mixed, kneaded, and allowed to rise, this bread dough would be turned into hot rolls for tonight and loaves of bread for three days.

This type of hot roll was almost always still warm about the time school was out. When matched with slices of vine-ripened tomatoes and nothing more than salt and pepper, these rolls, the odors and tastes would create childhood memories that would be remembered over and over again, silenced only by the grave.

Make bread for someone you love and give them something to remember, especially a child!

COMMON ERRORS IN BREAD MAKING

DEAD YEAST (Bread won't rise)

If warm water is good, then hot water must be better. Right? - Wrong! You just killed the yeast! Warm water means about the temperature of baby's milk (85 - 95 degrees F).

TOO MUCH FLOUR
The bread was kneaded too much and it just kept absorbing flour and more flour. The texture is course and the crust is hard.

OVER RISING

The dough tripled in size resulting in big air pockets and really irregular texture.

UNDER RISING

Bread that got cooked in the squat. As it was squatting to rise, you cooked it.

LOW OVEN TEMPERATURE

Very porous in center and upper half.

HIGH OVEN TEMPERATURE

Crust becomes very brown before bread has had a chance to cook.

KNEADING

Some recipes that follow are marked "easy to knead" and some are marked "hard to knead". The difference is entirely based upon the ratio of flour-to-liquid called for in the recipe.

Traditionally, three cups of flour when mixed with one cup of liquid will yield a dough that will not stick to your hands but is difficult for some petite people to knead into a fine load of bread. When the flour content is lowered to two cups, it takes well-floured hands to keep it from sticking. By lowering the amount of flour initially mixed with the liquid and adding flour around the sides, bottom, and top of the dough, it can be more easily turned into fine bread by a person who does not possess great strength and stamina.

Kneading is the act of pressing, stretching, and folding the dough, thereby separating the gluten and starch so that the bread will more readily hold its "rise" during the baking stage. A well kneaded loaf will be more uniform in size and texture. When dough ball becomes smooth and elastic and I'm tired of kneading, I stop. The dough always turns into bread and I always enjoy it, so don't worry if you have kneaded it long enough.

CARE OF BREAD JUST OUT OF THE OVEN

Remove bread from pans immediately after baking. Allow air to circulate all around the loaves. This will retain moisture. Allow to thoroughly cool before wrapping in plastic wrap. For a tender crust, cover hot bread with cloth.

YEAST BREADS

The yeast breads are broke down into three categories: first, standard yeast bread; second, salt-rising bread; third sour dough bread. This is a separation according to the type of yeast used in the bread.

THE STARTERS

STANDARD YEAST STARTER

1   packet rapid rise yeast
1   cup warm (85 - 95 degrees F) water
1   teaspoon sugar

Combine and allow yeast to dissolve for 5 or 10 minutes.

This yeast is a commercial strain available in any super market.

SALT RISING BREAD STARTER

1   medium potato, grated
1 1/2   cup boiling water
3   tablespoons corn meal
2   teaspoons sugar or honey
1   teaspoon salt

Random yeast or 1 packet rapid rise yeast. (If you want to try random yeast, just mix, cover, and wait to ferment; if you want the flavor, but just can't wait, just add yeast.)

Peel and grate potato and in a medium bowl, add to the boiling water, cornmeal, sugar, and salt. Allow to cool and stir in yeast. Cover and allow to set overnight. Warning: Do not add yeast to hot water!

SOUR DOUGH STARTER

Purchase a commercial starter or use the following recipe and allow to "sour" over time. It won't be San Francisco, but it works.

1   packet yeast (lager beer yeast preferred) (see note below)
2 1/2   cups luke-warm (85 - 95 degrees F) water
2   cups flour
1/4   cup sugar

Dissolve yeast in water, add sugar and flour, stir well and allow to sit for at least 24 hours. Stir every day. Note: Brewer "Lager" yeast was probably originally used and can be purchased from a local home-brew store.

All three of these starters can be maintained over a period of years simply by replacing original ingredients as they are used. For example, if you use a cup of sour dough starter, put a cupful of flour/water/sugar mixture back into your starter pot. Some strains, in fact, have been maintained for hundreds of years.

THE SPONGE

After you have a starter and you want to make bread, the most reliable method is to create a sponge. All you are really doing is allowing the yeast in your starter to multiply in an anaerobic environment (under water). This usually is accomplished overnight and results in a bowl of flour and water that has the appearance of a sponge. If it isn't frothing and full of holes (except for sour dough), then your yeast probably isn't any good and you will have to start over. The holes in the batter are caused by the rising and escaping carbon dioxide gas. This will provide "Leaven" for your bread. This gas, along with alcohol, are by-products formed by the single-celled yeast fungi as they devour, through fermentation, the sugars present in the act of multiplying. Alcohol you say! Yes, alcohol. Look at the ingredient lists for beer and for bread.

BEER	**BREAD**
Grain	Grain
Water	Water
Yeast	Yeast

By-products

BEER	BREAD
Carbon Dioxide Gas	Carbon Dioxide Gas
Alcohol	Alcohol

They are identical. In beer, the carbon dioxide gas provides the carbonation, whereas in bread, it provides bubbles that cause the bread to rise.

The alcohol in beer acts as a preservative and makes you tipsy. In bread, the alcohol is boiled off during baking and provides, in part, the distinctive odor of baking bread. If you were to capture the boiled-off alcohol and cool it (or distill it), you would have grain alcohol.

THE FLOURS

ALL-PURPOSE FLOUR

A white flour which contains satisfactory gluten for all types of baking. Gluten in wheat flour possesses properties which enable the dough to stretch and hold its shape during "leavening"

ENRICHED FLOUR

Vitamins and minerals added to all-purpose flour.

BLEACHED FLOUR

Processed by bleaching in order to have a whiter product. This changes the color of the flour, but adds nothing to the quality.

WHOLE WHEAT OR GRAHAM FLOUR

Made from the whole kernel of wheat containing varying amounts of bran and wheat germ. Makes for a coarser bread. Almost always used in conjunction with white flour.

RYE FLOUR

Rye is a hardy annual cereal grass, the flour of which is also almost always used in conjunction with white flour.

SELF-RISING FLOUR

An all-purpose flour containing baking powder and salt. This flour provides its own "leavening".

BREAD FLOUR (better for)

A white flour with a high gluten content; i.e. high protein.

CORN MEAL FLOUR

Ground corn containing no gluten.

STANDARD RECIPE FOR WHITE BREAD
HARD TO KNEAD - MAKES TWO 1-POUND LOAVES

1	packet rapid rise yeast
1/4	cup luke warm (85 - 95 degrees F) water
2	tablespoons sugar
1	teaspoon salt
2	cups non-fat skim milk (canned evaporated is okay)
6	cups unbleached flour
	Vegetable spray
	Corn meal

Add yeast, water, sugar and allow to dissolve for 5 to 10 minutes. Yeast should become active and bubbly the longer it sits. Pour into a large mixing pan along with the milk and salt. Stir and add 3 cups of flour. Add enough of the remaining flour to form into a soft dough ball. Knead, using remaining flour to deep dough from becoming sticky, until dough is firm and elastic. Place dough in veggie-sprayed bowl and allow to rise to about double its original size. Punch down, deflate and form into two loaves. Place in veggie-sprayed, cornmeal dusted, loaf pans or medium dutch oven. Cover and allow to rise to double original size. Preheat oven to 375 degrees F. Bake for 45 minutes. Remove and cool.

BASIC FRENCH BREAD OR ROLLS

HARD TO KNEAD - MAKES TWO SMALL LOAVES

1	package rapid rise yeast
1/4	cup warm (85 - 95 degrees F) water
1/2	teaspoon sugar
3	cups flour for bread or unbleached all-purpose flour
2	teaspoons salt
3/4	cup tap water
	Vegetable spray
	Cornmeal

Dissolve yeast in 1/4 cup warm water with sugar and let sit for 5 minutes. Add salt to liquid. In large mixing pan, combine with flour and rest of water. Work into a dough ball and knead. Add more flour to bottom and sides of pan to keep dough from sticking. Knead for 5 to 10 minutes or until dough ball becomes elastic, that is, resists being flattened out and folded over. Remove dough to a veggie-sprayed bowl that will hold dough after it has risen to twice its size. Cover bowl and allow to rise to double its size (about 50 to 60 minutes). This rising should take place in a warm (room temperature) place. After dough has risen, remove from bowl and punch it down or deflate it. Fold dough over end to end, put it back in veggie-sprayed bowl to rise again to double its original size. On floured counter top, press dough out into a 1/2-inch thick rectangle and with a knife, cut dough in half lengthwise. Fold sides of dough together, press inward and roll into a cigar-shaped loaf with your hands and rotate "cigar" back and forth to firm loaf, pinching the ends to seal loaf. Place on a veggie-sprayed, cornmeal dusted, cookie sheet, cover with clean towel and allow to rise to double its original size. Preheat oven to 450 degrees F. With a razor blade or sharp knife, make three diagonal slashes across top of loaves. Place loaves in oven and toss in five or six ice cubes into the bottom of the oven. This will create steam for a crunchy crust. Add four more ice cubes after five minutes. Lower temperature to 400 degrees F and bake for 30 minutes. Remove and allow to cool where air can get to all sides of the bread.

QUICK YEASTY DINNER BISCUITS
EASY TO KNEAD - MAKES ONE PIE PAN FULL

2/3	cup warm water
1	package rapid rise yeast (1/4 oz)
1 1/2	cup flour
1	teaspoon salt

Preheat oven to 400 degrees F. In large mixing bowl, dissolve yeast in warm water (85 to 95 degrees F). Add flour, salt and mix and form into a ball. Add more flour to the bottom of the pan to deep dough from being sticky and knead dough for five minutes. In bottom of mixing pan, press dough into a circle 1/4-inch thick. Using a small cookie cutter, cut dough into biscuits and place into a veggie-sprayed cake or pie pan. Cover pan with a clean dish towel and place on back of stove for 30 minutes. Uncover rolls and place in oven on medium high shelf and bake for 25 minutes.

POTATO-OATMEAL BREAD

EASY TO KNEAD - MAKES TWO LOAVES

2	cups hot non-fat milk
1	package yeast dissolved in 1/4 cup warm water and 1 tablespoon sugar and allowed to sit for 10 minutes
2	teaspoons salt
2	tablespoons sugar
1/2	cup instant mashed potato granules
1	cup regular oats
5	cups flour approximately
	Cornmeal

Mix yeast, water, and sugar and allow to sit for ten minutes. Mix hot milk, salt, sugar, potatoes, and oats. Allow to cool. Add the yeast solution and mix well. Add three cups of flour and mix; add one more cup and mix. Turn dough out onto a well-floured board or counter top and knead for a couple of minutes. Let dough rest for ten minutes. Knead dough until smooth and elastic, adding flour as needed to keep dough from being sticky. Place dough in large veggie-sprayed pan, cover and allow to rise to about double its original size. Punch down and form into two loaves and place in veggie-sprayed loaf pans, that have been dusted with corn meal. Cover and allow to rise until double in bulk. Bake in preheated 425 degree oven for ten minutes, reduce heat to 375 degrees and bake for 35 minutes more. Remove from pans and allow to cool. Note: for Pearl Barley bread, add two cups of barley that has been boiled for 15 minutes, and add another cup of flour.

WHOLE WHEAT BATTER BREAD
NO KNEADING REQUIRED
MAKES TWO SMALL LOAVES

2	cups luke-warm non-fat milk
1/4	cup molasses
1 1/2	teaspoon salt
1	package dry yeast
1/4	cup luke-warm water
4 1/3	cups whole wheat flour

Stir the yeast in the 1/4 cup luke-warm water and let it stand for five minutes to dissolve. Mix the milk, molasses, and salt in a large mixing bowl. Add the dissolved yeast and flour and beat well. Cover mixture with a clean towel and let rise in a warm place until double in size. Beat again briefly and put mixture into veggie-sprayed loaf pans. Cover and let rise to just less than double size. Preheat oven to 375 degrees. Bake bread for about 45 minutes. Remove from pan and cool.

SINGLE-RISE WHITE BREAD
EASY TO KNEAD
MAKES TWO LOAVES

1	teaspoon salt
1/2	cup sugar
2 1/4	cups luke-warm non-fat milk
1	package dry yeast
6	cups white flour

Mix everything but the flour in large mixing bowl and let sit for five minutes. Add three cups flour and beat until well blended. Add two more cups flour, mix, and place on well floured board or counter top. Add flour so dough is not sticky. Knead for five minutes, then let dough sit for ten minutes. From dough into two loaves and place in two veggie-sprayed loaf pans. Cover and let rise in warm place until dough doubles in size. Preheat oven to 425 degrees. Bake bread for ten minutes, reduce heat to 375 degrees for 25 minutes more. Remove from pans and cool.

WHOLE WHEAT BREAD
EASY TO KNEAD
MAKES TWO LOAVES

2	cups luke-warm non-fat milk
1	package dry yeast
1/4	cup sugar
2	teaspoons salt
2	cups whole-wheat flour
4	cups white flour
	Vegetable spray

Mix yeast and warm milk together and let stand for five minutes. Add sugar and salt and mix. Add two cups whole-wheat flour and two cups white flour. Mix thoroughly and pour out onto well-floured board or counter top, adding enough flour so that the dough isn't sticky. Knead for three or four minutes and then let sit for ten minutes. Resume kneading for about ten minutes, adding more white flour if dough is sticky. Place in veggie-sprayed bowl. Cover and let rise in a warm place until double in size. Polk down dough and form into two loaves or one loaf and a pan of rolls. Cover and let double in size. Preheat oven to 375 degrees and bake for about 40 minutes. Remove and cool on racks.

HONEY GRAHAM BREAD
EASY TO KNEAD
MAKES TWO SMALL LOAVES

1	cup salt rising or yeast starter from page 239
1	cup graham flour
1	tablespoon sugar
3 1/2	cups unbleached white flour
1	teaspoon imitation butter flavor
1	cup warm water (85 - 95 degrees F)
1	teaspoon salt
1/4	cup honey
	Vegetable spray
	Corn meal

The night before, in mixing bowl, combine starter, graham flour, 1 cup white flour, butter flavor, warm water, sugar, and salt. Stir, cover, and set in warm spot. The next day, combine with two cups white flour and form into dough ball. Use the rest of the flour when kneading bread for ten minutes to keep dough from sticking. Use more flour if necessary. Place dough in veggie-sprayed dish or pan, cover, and allow to rise to double in size. Punch down and place in veggie-sprayed dutch oven or baking pan that has been dusted with cornmeal. Bake in 350 degrees F preheated oven for 45 minutes. Remove and cool.

OATMEAL RAISIN GRAHAM BREAD
EASY TO KNEAD
MAKES ONE ROUND LOAF

1	cup starter (sour dough or salt rising from page 239)
1	cup uncooked oatmeal
1/2	cup raisins
2	tablespoons molasses or brown sugar
1	cup warm water (85 - 95 degrees F)
1	cup unbleached white bread flour
1 1/2	cup graham flour
	Cornmeal
	Vegetable spray

The night before, except for the graham flour, combine all ingredients, cover, and allow to sit all night. The next day, in large mixing bowl, combine with graham flour, form into a dough ball, and knead for ten minutes. Sprinkle on more graham flour in order to manage dough while kneading. Place dough in veggie-sprayed bowl, cover and allow to rise to double its size in a warm (not hot) spot. Punch down and place in round 8-inch oven pan that has been veggie-sprayed and cornmeal dusted. Dust top of bread with corn meal. Preheat oven to 375 degrees F and bake for 45 minutes.

SWEDISH LIMPA BREAD

MODERATE KNEAD
MAKES ONE LOAF

1	cup rye flour
2	cups unbleached bread flour
1	teaspoon anise seeds
1	package rapid rise yeast
2	tablespoons sugar
1	teaspoon salt
1	can evaporated skim milk
1	tablespoon molasses
2	tablespoons imitation butter flavoring
	Veggie spray
1	egg white, beaten slightly

In large mixing bowl, combine rye flour, bread flour, and anise seeds and mix. In small bowl, combine yeast, sugar, salt, milk, molasses, and butter flavoring. Mix thoroughly and pour into flour mixture. Form into a ball, add more bread flour around ball in order to facilitate kneading for ten minutes. Veggie spray another bowl or pan and place the round ball of dough in, cover, and allow to rise until double in size (about one hour). Punch down dough and form into a 14-inch long loaf with tapering ends. Place on veggie-sprayed cookie sheet, cover, and let rise again to double its size. Preheat oven to 400 degrees F. With a sharp knife or razor, make 5 slashes across loaf about 1/4 inch deep and brush loaf with egg white. Place in oven, reduce temperature to 375 degrees F, and bake for 30 minutes until loaf sounds hollow when tapped.

SURE-FIRE SALT-RISIN' BREAD

This bread is yet another effort to put air bubbles in bread dough. Without a rising agent, flour dough ends up hard, gloppy, and unappetizing.

Originally, this starter relied upon luck in finding a random, wandering yeast culture, whether airborne or coexisting with the potato, corn meal, or sugar. Probably, unpasteurized, wild honey would have been more useful than the sugar in providing a source of random yeast.

Once the random yeast is combined with the sugar, potato, and cornmeal, it begins to devour the sugars and multiply.

This form of spontaneous fermentation was at best unreliable. To insure a reliable rising agent, we simply add to our starter a packet of rapid rise dry yeast. Incidentally, the salt was thought to improve and guarantee results.

This recipe makes two 8-inch loaves.

SALT-RISIN' STARTER

1	medium or 2 small potatoes
1 1/2	cup boiling water
3	tablespoons corn meal
2	teaspoons sugar or honey
1	teaspoon salt
1	packet rapid rise yeast

Peel and shred the potato and, in a medium bowl, add to the water, cornmeal, sugar, and salt. Allow to cool and stir in the yeast. Cover and allow to sit overnight.

Now this mixture is going to begin to ferment, forming by-products of carbon dioxide gas and alcohol. As this occurs, the yeast multiplies.

The next day, you have a soupy, goopy mixture which is very rich in yeast and alcohol. For those whose lips never touch alcohol, not to fear, it will all boil off during the baking process. This alcohol occurs during the making of all yeast breads. Stir and strain off one cup of the liquid, putting the solids back into the bowl.

Now lets make some of the most delicious bread you have ever tasted.

THE SALT-RISIN' BREAD DOUGH
MODERATE KNEAD
MAKES TWO LOAVES

1	cup starter liquid from previous page
1	packet rapid rise yeast
6	cups all-purpose flour
1/4	teaspoon baking soda
1	cup non-fat, evaporated, skim milk
1	egg white

Mix yeast into starter liquid and allow to dissolve. In a large mixing bowl, combine flour, baking soda, milk, and starter liquid. Stir until well mixed, knead for five to ten minutes until smooth. Add more flour if necessary to manage. Using veggie spray, lightly grease two 8-inch loaf pans. Divide dough into two parts, shape into loaves, and place in loaf pans. With sharp knife, make several diagonal cuts across tops of loaves - about 1/4-inch deep. Set loaves on top of stove, cover with a dish towel, and allow to rise to double their size (about one hour). Preheat oven to 375 degrees F. After bread has risen, brush tops with egg white and place on medium rack in oven and bake for 35 minutes until golden brown and loaf sounds hollow when tapped. Remove from oven and allow to cool on top of stove for 10 minutes; remove from pans and allow to cool somewhat. While still warm, slice off one end piece and with a very fresh cup of coffee, sit down, kick back, and enjoy the fruits of your honest labor.

SALT-RISIN' OATMEAL RAISIN BREAD
EASY TO KNEAD
MAKES ONE 9-INCH ROUND, 4-INCH HIGH LOAF

1	cup liquid starter from page 239
1	cup uncooked oatmeal
2 1/2	cups flour for bread
1	cup warm water
	Vegetable spray
	Cornmeal

The night before, combine starter, oatmeal, one cup flour, and warm water. Stir, cover with plastic wrap, and let rest overnight. The next day, add one cup flour and stir to form into a dough ball. Sprinkle a part of the remaining flour on top of and around dough. Knead for five minutes and place in veggie-sprayed dish or pan. Cover and allow to rise to double its size. Punch down, form into a load and place in a veggie-sprayed pan that has been dusted with cornmeal. Brush or sprinkle top of dough with warm water and sprinkle cornmeal on top. Preheat oven to 375 degrees F, when dough has almost risen to double its original size, bake for 45 minutes. Remove from pan and allow to cool.

SALT-RISIN' BREAKFAST BISCUITS (WHITE FLOUR)
EASY TO KNEAD
MAKES ONE 10" PAN OF BISCUITS

Prepare the night before use.

1/2	cup starter liquid from page 239
1/2	cup evaporated skim milk or reconstituted non-fat powdered milk
1/2	teaspoon salt
2	cups all-purpose flour

In a large, stainless steel mixing pan, combine ingredients and form into a ball. Add more flour as needed in order to manage the dough. It shouldn't stick to your hands as you knead the dough for 5 to 7 minutes. In the bottom of the mixing pan, press out the dough until the size of a 9- or 10-inch cake pan. Cut biscuits and place in veggie-sprayed cake pan or other oven-proof pan. Cover with plastic wrap and sit on top of stove overnight. The next morning, preheat oven to 400 degrees F and bake for 20 minutes until golden brown.

BREAKFAST SALT-RISIN' CINNAMON RAISIN ROLLS

1/2	cup starter liquid from page 239
1/2	cup evaporated skim milk
1	teaspoon vanilla, butter, nut flavoring
1/2	teaspoon salt (optional)
2	cups all-purpose flour
1/2	cup raisins
1/2	cup brown sugar (loosely packed)
1	teaspoon cinnamon
	Vegetable spray

The night before, in a large stainless steel mixing pan, combine and mix starter liquid, milk, flavoring, salt, and flour. Mix well into a ball and knead for 5 to 10 minutes adding more flour as needed to manage. Turn dough onto a floured surface and roll into a 1/8-inch thick rectangular shape. Sprinkle cinnamon, sugar, and raisins evenly over the entire surface. Roll dough up into a giant burrito-like shape. Cut roll into 1/2- to 3/4-inch thick sections and place flat side down in a veggie-sprayed 9-inch cake pan or equivalent. Cover well and let sit overnight. The next morning, place in 400 degrees F preheated oven for 20 minutes until golden brown. Serve warm. Freeze leftovers.

SALT-RISING WAFFLES OR GRIDDLE CAKES
FOR TWO

1/2	cup salt-rising starter liquid from page 239
1	cup all-purpose flour
1	teaspoon baking powder
1	tablespoon sugar (optional)
2	moderately beaten egg whites
	Vegetable spray

In mixing bowl, combine flour, sugar, and baking powder. Mix thoroughly. Add beaten eggs and starter liquid and beat gently until batter is smooth. Pour batter into hot veggie-sprayed waffle iron or griddle. Enjoy.

SALT-RISIN' TEA BREAD
MAKES SIX HAMBURGER BUN SIZE ROLLS

1	packet rapid rise yeast

1	cup starter liquid from page 239
1	teaspoon imitation butter flavoring
1	tablespoon sugar (optional)
2	cups unbleached all-purpose bread flour
	Vegetable spray

Preheat oven to 425 degrees F. Combine starter liquid, butter flavoring, yeast, and sugar. Dissolve yeast, then combine with flour. Form into a ball and knead for 5 to 10 minutes until dough is springy and elastic. Divide dough into 3 x 3/4-inch biscuits and place on a veggie-sprayed cookie sheet. Cover and in a warm spot, allow to rise until double in size. Put in oven and bake for 20 minutes until golden brown. Allow to cool, then slice very thing and serve with jam or preserves.

SALT-RISIN' BUTTER COCONUT STICKY BUNS
MAKES TWELVE

2	cups unbleached flour
2	tablespoons sugar
1	cup salt-risin' starter liquid from page 239
2	teaspoons liquid imitation butter flavoring
1	teaspoon imitation coconut extract
1/2	cup raisins
1	cup brown sugar
2	teaspoons cinnamon
	Vegetable spray

Prepare the night before. Mix starter liquid with coconut flavor and butter flavor. In a mixing bowl, combine flour and sugar, then add starter/flavor mixture. From into a ball and knead for 10 minutes, adding more flour to make dough manageable. Roll out dough to rectangle about 3/8-inch thick. Spread on brown sugar, raisins, and cinnamon. Roll up in a tight pin wheel, cut 1/2-inch thick slices and place each in veggie-sprayed muffin tin. Cover and allow to rise all night. the next morning, preheat oven to 400 degrees F and bake for 15 to 20 minutes. Remove and serve warm.

SALT-RISIN' PUMPKIN BREAD
MAKES ONE 9-INCH LOAF

1/2	cup salt risin' liquid from page 239
1	cup canned pumpkin
1	teaspoon pumpkin pie spice
4	tablespoons sugar
1/2	cup raisins
2	cups unbleached bread flour
	Vegetable spray

In the evening, in a large mixing bowl combine salt risin' liquid, pumpkin, spice, sugar, and raisins. Mix well, then add flour and form into a ball. Add more flour around ball of dough and knead for 7 to 10 minutes. From into a loaf and place into a 9-inch loaf pan. Cover with dish towel and allow to rise all night. The next morning, preheat oven to 350 degrees F and bake loaf for 40 to 45 minutes until loaf is golden brown and sounds hollow when tapped on top. Slice warm for a nice breakfast, brunch, or tea bread.

SALT-RISIN' SIMPLE BREAKFAST MUFFINS
MAKES TWELVE MUFFINS

2	cups unbleached flour
1	cup starter liquid from page 239
1/2	cup evaporated milk
2	tablespoons sugar

1/2   cup raisins
2   tablespoons oat bran
        Vegetable spray

The night before, mix ingredients until smooth and spoon into a veggie-sprayed muffin tin. Cover and allow to rise overnight. The next morning, preheat oven to 400 degrees F and bake for 25 minutes.

SALT-RISIN' EGG BREAD
EASY TO KNEAD - MAKES TWO ROUND 6-INCH LOAVES 3 INCHES HIGH

1   cup starter liquid from page 239
1   packet rapid rise yeast
1/2   cup Egg Beaters® egg substitute
2 1/2   cups unbleached flour
1   tablespoon oat bran
        (optional but recommended)
1   slightly beaten egg white
        Vegetable spray

Preheat oven to 400 degrees F. Dissolve yeast in starter liquid and mix in bowl with the flour and egg substitute. Form into a ball, pour more flour around dough and knead for 5 to 10 minutes. Divide dough in half and form into round balls. Place separated on a veggie-sprayed cookie sheet. Cover loaves, place on top of stove and allow to rise until double in size (about 1 hour). Using a sharp knife or razor blade slash each loaf 2 or 3 times about 1/4 inch deep. Brush completely with egg whites and place in oven. Lower heat to 375 degrees F and bake for 30 minutes.

SALT-RISIN' BAGELS

Preheat oven to 375 degrees F. Use dough from Salt-Risin' Bread on page 252 or other bread dough recipe and one beaten egg white. After dough has risen to double its size, punch down and form into 3-inch disks (about the size of a donut). Poke a 1-inch hole in middle and form into bagel. Place on veggie-sprayed cookie sheet, cover, and allow to rise again to about double size (30 to 40 minutes). Bring a pan of water to a boil and immerse a bagel into water and turn over immediately. Immediately remove bagel with a slotted spoon or spatula and place on veggie-sprayed surface to drain. Place bagels on veggie-sprayed cookie sheet, brush with egg white, and bake for 20 minutes until golden brown. Freeze leftover bagels.

SOUR DOUGH BREAD

Sour dough and beans have been almost inseparable ever since there has been sour dough. So for that reason, I have left them together here in the "Bread" chapter. It might seem a little weird to find a bean recipe in amongst the breads, but I assure you that they really are partners.

SMOKEY RANCH BEANS AND SOUR DOUGH BISCUITS

A hundred years ago, on a western cattle drive, you could always count on the blackened bean pot (usually cast iron) to be filled in the morning with beans and water and allowed to slush around aboard the chuck wagon all day long. After the evening meal, the bean pot was placed next to the campfire and allowed to simmer most of the night. Chopped up bits and pieces of leftover, fire-grilled beef along with a little sugar, and salt were added to the pot and perhaps some onions or molasses if available. Wild onions were and are readily available over much of the old western cattle drive country. After the beans were beginning their all-night affair with the camp fire, the sour dough starter was opened and a portion of this liquid starter was poured into the biscuit making pan. Warm water from the water barrel strapped to the side of the chuck wagon and some flour was added to the starter so as to make a thick liquid. This liquid was allowed to sit while clean-up chores were attended to. What happened in the bread pan during the next several hours largely determined the overall success or failure of the cook. Should the sourdough fail, then baking powder biscuits would be the back up bread, however, yeast bread was always preferred. A good cook could make good bread, everything else was second fiddle.

The first step in the sour dough biscuit process was simply to add more flour, some salt, knead, and form into biscuit balls. These dough balls were placed in a big dutch oven, covered, and set aside to begin their all-night rising effort. The next morning, when placed next to the campfire, these rolls were soon baked into golden goodness and when matched with the bubbly, beefy beans, they provided really substantial food. This low-fat fare, when washed down with plenty of hot cowboy coffee, would keep a person going all day long.

SMOKEY RANCH BEANS

2   cups small dry white beans
1   cup burnt end pieces of beef
      (well browned trimmings) or meat
      from 1 Pit Bar-B-Que Beef sandwich
4   cups water
1   small onion
1/2   teaspoon salt
1/4   cup brown sugar
1/3   cup molasses

Clean and soak beans all night, drain water prior to combining ingredients. Remove all visible fat from beef and chop into small pieces. Place beef in a dutch oven (or big pot) along with four cups of water and boil vigorously for 1/2 hour or so. Remove from heat and skim off any surface grease. Add onion, salt, sugar, and beans, and simmer until beans are tender and the juice is thick. Add more hot water to cooking beans as needed. Remove from heat and serve. Beans are more flavorful the second and third day.

Note: Some would add 1/4 cup of bar-b-que sauce or plain tomato sauce. I believe this alters the authenticity, but it also tastes good.

SOUR DOUGH BISCUITS

1   cup sour dough starter from page 239
5   cups flour
1   cup water
1   teaspoon salt
      Vegetable spray

Preheat oven to 375 degrees F. In a large mixing bowl, combine starter, water, salt, and 1 cup of flour. Stir this soupy mixture well, cover, and allow to rest and rise in a warm place (but not hot!). After a couple of hours, the mixture should be an active, bubbly bee hive of yeasty proliferation. Add rest of flour, stir, and form into a ball. Add more flour over dough, as needed, and knead for 10 minutes. Divide dough into golf-ball size pieces and place side by side in a veggie-sprayed dutch oven or cast iron skillet. Cover and allow to rise until the biscuits double in size. Bake for 40 minutes or until golden brown and hollow sounding when thumped. Serve hot from the oven.

BASIC SOUR DOUGH BREAD
HARD TO KNEAD
MAKES 1 BIG ROUND OR 2 SMALL LOAVES

1	cup starter from page 239
1	cup water
2	teaspoons salt
2	tablespoons sugar
5 1/2	cups flour
	Vegetable spray
	Cornmeal

The night before mix starter, water, 1 cup flour, salt, and sugar. Stir well, cover, and allow to sit all night. The next day, in a large mixing pan, combine frothy, foamy starter mixture that has been sitting all night with 4 1/2 cups of flour. Stir, forming into a ball of dough, knead for 10 minutes or until dough is smooth and elastic. Place dough in a veggie-sprayed pan or bowl that will allow sufficient room for the dough to rise to double its size. After doubling in size, punch down, and form into loaf or loaves and place in veggie-sprayed, cornmeal dusted baking pan or pans. Preheat oven to 375 degrees F. After dough has risen to double its original size, place in oven and bake for 40 minutes or until loaf is browned, sounds hollow when tapped, and has shrunk away from the sides of the pan. Remove and cool on wire rack.

SOUR DOUGH OATMEAL RAISIN BREAD
EASY TO KNEAD
MAKES TWO SMALL LOAVES

1	cup sour dough starter from page 239
1	cup warm water (85 to 95 degrees F)
1	cup dry, rolled oats - regular or quick
2 1/2	cups unbleached flour
1	cup raisins
1	teaspoon salt
	Vegetable spray
1	tablespoon cornmeal

The night before, combine starter, water, rolled oats, 1 cup flour, raisins, and salt. Stir well, cover with plastic wrap, and allow to rest all night. The next day, add and mix 1 cup flour and knead for five minutes. Use remaining 1/2 cup flour to dust on and around dough to keep it from sticking. Place in a veggie-sprayed dutch oven or other oven-proof cookware, cover, and allow to rise to double its size. Punch down and dust top with cornmeal; allow to rise again to almost double its original size. Preheat oven to 375 degrees F and bake for 45 minutes. Remove and allow to cool somewhat.

LAGER BREAD

HARD TO KNEAD
MAKES ONE LARGE ROUND OR TWO SMALL
LOAVES

1	cup sour dough lager starter from page 239
	(sour dough starter made with lager yeast)
1	cup water
2	teaspoons salt
1	tablespoon sugar
5 1/2	cups flour
	Vegetable spray
	Corn meal

The night before, in a mixing bowl, combine and stir thoroughly starter, water, salt, sugar, and 1 cup flour. Cover with plastic wrap and allow to sit over night. The next day, in a large mixing pan, add 4 1/2 cups of flour and starter mixture. Form into a ball and knead until smooth and elastic. Place in veggie-sprayed pan, cover with plastic wrap, and allow to rise to double its original size in a warm (75 to 80 degrees F) spot. Punch down and form into a loaf or loaves and place in a veggie-sprayed, cornmeal-dusted pan. Preheat oven to 375 degrees F. When dough has risen to double its original size, place in oven and bake for 40-45 minutes until brown, hollow sounding when thumped, and somewhat shrunken away from sides of the pan. Remove from oven and take bread immediately from pans and allow to cool on a wire rack where air can get to all sides of the bread.

QUICK BREADS

A s the name implies, these breads require much less time to prepare. They do not use yeast as a leavening agent, instead they rely upon a chemical reaction to create carbon dioxide gas, the built-in air from beaten eggs or steam. They include biscuits, muffins, crumpets, cornbread, steamed breads, popovers, griddle cakes, waffles, and Irish soda bread. With the exception of Irish soda bread, they are almost always served hot.

BAKING POWDER - BAKING SODA

When you combine an acid with bicarbonate of soda, you produce a large quantity of carbon dioxide gas which makes your dough fluff up or rise. Baking soda is a bicarbonate of soda, which is the main ingredient of baking powder. Sour cream, yogurt, vinegar, or sour milk are very acid and react quickly with baking soda.

POPOVERS
MAKES SIX

1/2	cup nonfat skim milk
1/4	cup Egg Beaters® egg substitute
1/2	cup flour
1	tablespoon Butter Buds® butter flavor granules
1/8	teaspoon salt
	Vegetable spray

Preheat oven to 450 degrees F. Spray non-stick muffin tin with butter flavored vegetable spray. Beat eggs for a minute or two, add rest of ingredients and mix thoroughly. Spoon mixture into six muffins and place in oven. After 15 minutes, lower temperature to 350 degrees F. DO NOT OPEN OVEN UNTIL 15 MORE MINUTES HAVE ELAPSED. Serve immediately with your favorite topping or use as bread. To make 12 popovers, just double the ingredients.

QUICK FAT-FREE FLOUR TORTILLAS

1   package of generic biscuit dough
       (1 gram of fat per 2 biscuits)
    OR
1   package of french bread dough
       (1 gram of fat per slice or less)

On well floured board or counter top, combine 2 biscuits into a ball. roll in flour, then roll out the size of a tortilla. Turn dough, adding flour to top frequently. Place tortilla into medium hot skillet. Turn when dough starts to puff up. Remove when tortilla is spotted with dark brown spots. Don't overcook. Remove to plate and cover with plastic wrap.

SOUR CREAM BISCUITS

2   cups self-rising flour
1   tablespoon Butter Buds® butter
       flavoring granules
1   teaspoon cheddar cheese sprinkles
       (optional)
1   cup sour cream from page 321
       Vegetable spray

Preheat oven to 425 degrees F. In mixing bowl combine and mix the flour, butter flavor, and cheese sprinkles. Add sour cream, mix, and form into a ball. Add more flour around ball and knead for 2 or 3 minutes. Press into a 1/2-inch thick oval and then, using a cookie cutter or glass, cut dough into biscuits and place on a veggie-sprayed pan, keeping them separated. Bake for 20 minutes until done.

VARIATIONS OF SOUR CREAM BISCUITS

CHEESE SANDWICH BISCUIT

Roll or press dough to 1/4-inch thickness; cut into biscuits, place slightly smaller piece of fat-free cheese on bottom piece, and place another biscuit on top and press edges together. You now have a 1/2-inch thick biscuit with a piece of cheese in the middle.

HAM AND CHEESE BISCUIT
Add sliced ham pieces to cheese middle.

PINEAPPLE BISCUIT
Place one biscuit on bottom; cut a 1-inch hole in another biscuit and place on top. Fill hole with pineapple jelly. Other flavors optional.

MEAT AND POULTRY FILLING
Make bottom biscuit thinner, cut 1-inch hole in thicker top biscuit and leave empty. After cooking, fill with a favorite spread.

FRESH FRUIT FILLING

Prepare as per meat and poultry filling except substitute fresh fruit and top with cheese cake topping.

QUICK IRISH SODA BREAD

4   cups self-rising flour
2   tablespoons sugar
1   cup raisins
2   cups buttermilk
     (reconstituted powdered buttermilk is fine)
     Vegetable spray
     Preheat oven to 375 degrees F

In mixing bowl, thoroughly mix flour and sugar. Add raisins and buttermilk, mix, and form into a ball. Knead for 5 minutes, form into a round loaf, and place on a veggie-sprayed baking sheet (or pan). Make two 1/2-inch deep cuts across loaf to form a cross and bake for 40 to 45 minutes until brown and sounds hollow when thumped on top. Remove from oven and allow to cool. Slice very thin, NEVER THICK. Makes great toast.

CHEESY IRISH SODA BREAD

     Irish soda bread from preceding recipe
2   tablespoons cheese flavored sprinkles

Omit raisins and 1 tablespoon of sugar from recipe and add 2 tablespoons of cheese flavored sprinkles. Prepare and bake as indicated.

IRISH SODA CINNAMON ROLLS

MAKES ONE 9-INCH CAKE PAN FULL

2   cups all-purpose unbleached flour
1/2   teaspoon baking soda
1/2   teaspoon baking powder
1/2   teaspoon salt

1   tablespoon sugar
1/2   cup raisins
1   cup buttermilk
1   teaspoon vanilla flavoring
1   teaspoon butter flavoring
THE FILLING
1   teaspoon cinnamon
1/2   cup brown sugar
        Vegetable spray

Preheat oven to 400 degrees F. In mixing bowl, mix thoroughly flour, soda, raisins, baking powder, salt, and sugar. Add flavorings to buttermilk (reconstituted powdered buttermilk works well) then combine buttermilk with flour mixture. Form into a ball, add more flour to manage dough, and knead for 5 minutes. Turn out onto floured surface, and press down into a 12 x 6 x 3/8-inch form. Sprinkle dough with brown sugar and cinnamon and roll up into a pinwheel. Slice into 3/4-inch thick rolls and place in a veggie-sprayed 9-inch cake pan. Bake for 20 minutes until golden brown. Serve warm.

IRISH SODA BREAD

4   cups all-purpose flour
        (unbleached if available)
1   teaspoon baking soda
1   teaspoon baking powder
1   teaspoon salt
2   tablespoons sugar
1   cup raisins
2   cups buttermilk
        Vegetable spray

Preheat oven to 375 degrees F. In large mixing bowl, mix thoroughly the flour, soda, baking powder, salt, and sugar. Then add raisins and buttermilk. form into a ball and knead for 5 minutes or so until smooth. Form into a round loaf and place on a veggie-sprayed sheet pan. With a sharp knife, cut a 1/2-inch deep cross on top of loaf. Bake for 40 to 45 minutes until nicely brown and sounds hollow when tapped on top. The cross will have spread into the characteristic trademark of Irish soda bread. Cool and slice thin. Makes wonderful toast.

STEWED IRISH SODA BREAD

Use the recipe for Irish soda bread substituting 1 1/2 cups (1 can) lite beer and 1/2 cup buttermilk for the 2 cups of buttermilk.

CHEDDAR CORN BREAD
MAKES ONE 9-INCH CAKE PAN

1	cup self-rising flour
1/2	cup corn meal
2	teaspoons cheddar flavored sprinkles
1	cup liquid buttermilk (reconstituted powder is okay)
	Vegetable spray

Preheat oven to 400 degrees F. In mixing bowl, mix thoroughly flour, corn meal, and cheddar sprinkles. Add buttermilk and mix well. Spoon out into cornbread molds or a veggie-sprayed 9-inch cake pan. Bake for 20 to 25 minutes. Serve warm.

HERBED CHEESE BISCUITS

2   cups self rising flour
1/4   teaspoon each of dried parsley, oregano, thyme, and marjoran
1   tablespoon Molly McButter® all natural cheese flavored sprinkles
2   teaspoons imitation butter flavor
1   cup evaporated skim milk
      Vegetable spray

Preheat oven to 450 degrees F. In a large mixing bowl, mix flour, herbs, and cheese sprinkles. In measuring cup, mix butter flavor and milk, then pour into flour. Stir and form into a ball. Add more flour around ball of dough and knead for 3 or 4 minutes. Press out into a 1/2- to 3/4-inch thick circle. Using cookie cutter, cut into biscuits and place apart on veggie-sprayed cookie sheet. Bake for 12 to 15 minutes.

VERY QUICK YEAST ROLLS

1   cup warm water (85-95 degrees)
1   package rapid rise yeast
1/4   cup sugar
2   cups self rising flour
1/4   cup nonfat milk powder
2   teaspoons vinegar
1   tablespoon skim milk
      Grated parmesian or Romano cheese
      Vegetable spray

Combine water, yeast, sugar and allow to sit at room temperature for at least 1/4 hour or until 1/2 inch of foam forms on top of liquid. Preheat oven to 400 degrees F. In large mixing pan combine flour and milk powder. Add vinegar to yeast liquid, stir well and pour into the flour. Mix into a dough ball and knead for 4 or 5 minutes. Sprinkle with more flour to facilitate kneading. Cut into biscuits and place in veggie sprayed 9" cake pan. Brush tops with skim milk and sprinkle with cheese. Allow to sit on top of stove for 10 minutes then bake for 20 minutes.

NOTE: For a butter-cheese flavored roll add 2 teaspoons imitation butter flavoring and 1 tablespoon Molly McButter® natural cheese flavor sprinkles. Your rolls will be a golden yellow color.

SOUR CREAM OR BUTTERMILK SCONES

2   cups self-rising flour
1   cup sour cream from page 321 or buttermilk
1   teaspoon vanilla, butter, nut flavoring
2   tablespoons sugar
1/2   cup raisins
       Vegetable spray

Preheat oven to 450 degrees F. Combine ingredients, stir, and form into a ball. Add more flour around dough so it doesn't stick to your hands as you knead the dough for 3 or 4 minutes. Flatten into a circle of dough about 1/2- to 3/4-inch thick. With biscuit or cookie cutter, cut into biscuits and place separated in a veggie-sprayed pan or cookie sheet. Bake for 15 to 20 minutes until golden brown and done. Serve warm for tea time with raspberry jam (grape will do).

SCONES

2   cups all-purpose flour (unbleached is best)
1   tablespoon baking powder
1/2   teaspoon salt
1   tablespoon sugar
1   cup evaporated skim milk
      Vegetable spray

Preheat oven to 450 degrees F. Combine and mix thoroughly flour, baking powder, salt, and sugar. Add milk and quickly stir mixture and form into a ball. Knead dough for 3 to 5 minutes, then pat out to a thickness of 1/2 inch. Cut into biscuits and place on veggie-sprayed cookie sheet or pan. Bake 12 to 15 minutes until golden brown.

BUTTERMILK PANCAKES

2 1/2 cups buttermilk either fresh or reconstituted dry buttermilk
1/2   cup Egg Beaters® egg substitute
1/2   teaspoon salt
1   teaspoon baking soda
3   cupfuls flour

Mix buttermilk, eggs, salt, and baking soda thoroughly. Add flour and beat until smooth. Do not over beat. Spoon onto veggie-sprayed hot griddle or pan and cook until top is full of holes and the underside in brown. Turn and brown other side. Batter should be used immediately after mixing. Leftover batter may be mixed with raisins and spooned into veggie-sprayed muffin tin and baked at 350 degrees F for 20 minutes or until done.

FRENCH TOAST

Thick slices of homemade bread are best for French toast. Thick slices of other bread are second best.

1/4	cup Egg Beaters® egg substitute
1	cup non-fat milk
	Dash nutmeg
	Dash cinnamon
1	tablespoon sugar

Mix well. Dip bread slices into mixture. Do not soak. Fry on hot veggie-sprayed griddle or skillet. Brown both sides, remove and sprinkle with powdered sugar.

FILLED FRENCH TOAST

With an unsliced loaf of bread, slice a 1/4- to 3/8-inch thick slice partially through the loaf (close to the bottom). Move knife over 1/4- to 3/8-inch and make another slice completely through the loaf. You should now have a thick slice of bread hinged at the bottom. Spread inside of slice (or pocket) with your favorite jam or jelly, dip in french toast batter and fry.

X. DESSERTS

When the sweet tooth craving strikes and you feel it has to be satisfied, at least do it without fat. This chapter will show you how.

The average American consumes approximately 128 pounds of sugar each year. The standard argument among the lay people, has always been that sugar has been shown to only cause cavities in your teeth and otherwise is not detrimental to your health. Right? Wrong!!

As long ago as 1986, it has been shown that elevated levels of triglycerides are a highly significant independent risk factor for coronary heart disease in women, according to William P. Castelli, M.D., Director of the famous Framingham Heart Study. (AM Heart Journal, Vol. 112, page 432, 1986) In addition, they appear important in men with low HDL cholesterol (the good guys). Individuals with elevated triglycerides should be considered at risk for coronary heart disease unless the total cholesterol/HDL ratio is under 3.5 (refer to Chapter 6). More recently, this same conclusion was reached by a group of Finnish researchers (See: Joint Effects of Serum Triglyceride and LDL cholesterol and HDL cholesterol concentration on coronary heart disease risk in the Helsinki Heart Study; January 1992, issue of circulation published by the American Heart Association: Circulation 1992; 85: 37-45) The Helsinki summary is, "The present data suggests that elevated serum triglyceride concentration is a marker of elevated coronary heart disease risk, especially in subjects with a high LDL/HDL ratio".

So what does all this have to do with sugar? Your liver converts excess calories from carbohydrates (as in sugar) first into fatty acids and then into triglycerides. The more excess sugar, the more elevated serum triglycerides.

Recently, I took advantage of a free cholesterol screening at the Lipid and Arteriosclerosis Prevention Clinic, Department of Medicine, Division of Clinical Pharmacology, University of Kansas Medical Center; located in Kansas City. Here are the results:

Total Cholesterol: 183 (good)
Triglycerides: 394 (terrible)
HDL: 25 (bad)
LDL: 79 (good)
Ratio LDL/HDL: 3.71 (good)

Since my triglycerides should have been less than 200, I was asked to come in for a second screening and was told, "by the way, I know you are writing the chapter in your book about desserts, so why don't you refrain from consuming excessive amounts of sugar" for two weeks prior, to the second screening. I gave up sugar and the results were as follows:

Total cholesterol: 188
Triglycerides: 153
HDL: 29
LDL: 128
Ratio LDL/HDL: 4.43

I had always been a big sugar eater with elevated triglyceride levels hovering around 400 and no one had ever proclaimed me at risk for coronary heart disease until the Lipid Clinic at the University of Kansas. Fortunately, they also prescribed a simple remedy, "Don't eat so much sugar", and it brought my triglyceride levels down where they belonged.

The moral of this story is MODERATION. Be moderate in your consumption of sugar and always take the fat out. Remember: There isn't a dime's worth of difference between sugars. If it's sweet, it's probably sugar and you can't rationalize a difference between juice concentrate, honey, brown sugar, or molasses. It is all sugar!

For your Thanksgiving Day dessert table, I recommend some or all of the following items with 1 gram of fat per serving or less. (With the exception of chocolate fudge cheesecake which has approximately 1.5 grams per serving):

-Pumpkin Pie, page 282
-Lemon Meringue Pie, page 281
-Cream Cheese, Maraschino Cherry
 Spread, page 102
 with Mini Loaves of Pumpkin Bread,
 page 257
-Raspberry Shortcake, page 302
-Pineapple Up-side-down Cake, page 298
-Olde, Olde Fashioned Cake, page 290
-Chocolate Fudge Cheese Cake, page 304

For your Christmas cookie selection, why not try some of the following with less than 1 gram of fat per cookie:

-Brownie Oatmeal, page 310
-Brown Sugar Raisin, page 309
-Brownies, page 306
-Chocolate Raisin, page 309
-Chocolate-Covered Cherry Cookies,
 page 308

Remember the key word when it comes to sugary desserts - MODERATION - and just no fat. Good luck!

PIE CRUSTS AND PIES

BISCUIT PIE CRUST
(REGULAR OR BUTTERMILK)

A traditional fat ladened pie crust has approximately 10 to 15 grams of fat per serving. This recipe, using a whole can of generic biscuits (10), will contain just 5 grams for the entire crust!

1   can biscuits (1 gram of fat per 2 biscuits)
2   tablespoons sugar
       Flour
       Vegetable spray

Remove biscuits to mixing bowl and sprinkle with sugar. Press in sugar and form biscuits into a dough ball. Remove to floured surface and roll into 12- to 14-inch circle. Place into a veggie-sprayed pie pan.

CAKE CRUMB PIE CRUST

One cup of graham cracker crumbs has approximately 14 grams of fat. Using two cups per pie would amount to about 5 grams of fat per serving in the crust alone.
The following crust yields 0 grams of fat per serving.

CHOCOLATE CAKE CRUMB CRUST

2   cups non-fat chocolate cake
       Water to moisten, if needed

In mixing bow, crumble cake and sprinkle lightly with water if needed. in veggie-sprayed pie pan, press crumbs to sides and bottom.

YELLOW CAKE CRUMB PIE CRUST

       Non-fat yellow cake or pound cake
       Water to moisten if needed.

Crumble cake and sprinkle lightly with water, if needed. In veggie-sprayed pie pan, press crumbs to the sides and bottom.

CORN FLAKE CRUMB CRUST

1   cup corn flake crumbs (buy them in a box
       or make them yourself)
2   tablespoons sugar
2   tablespoons water
       Vegetable spray

Thoroughly mix ingredients in a mixing bowl. Pour into a veggie-sprayed pie pan. Press and form to shape pie crust. Chill well before filling. Use where graham cracker crusts are called for. Chill before serving.

FLOUR TORTILLA PIE CRUST

Perhaps the easiest pie crust ever, is accomplished by taking a large flour tortilla, holding it under the hot water faucet for a few moments, laying in on a towel to dry a little, and then placing it in a pie pan. Each large tortilla generally has less than 5 grams of fat so it will provide a very low fat crust. If baking this crust empty, be sure to poke a few holes in the bottom and around the sides to deep large bubbles of air from forming. Use as you would any pie crust.

TWO CRUST PIE CRUST

2	cups self-rising flour
3/4	cup buttermilk
1/4	cup apple juice concentrate
1	teaspoon imitation butter flavoring
1	teaspoon vanilla flavoring
	Vegetable spray
1	egg white, beaten slightly

Combine buttermilk, apple juice concentrate, and flavorings. Pour into flour and form into a moist ball. Pour more self-rising flour around dough, then knead for 5 minutes. On a smooth, floured surface, roll out 2/3 of dough into circle about 1/8-inch thick. Place in a veggie-sprayed pie pan. Trim edges, poke fork holes in the bottom, and place in a 350 degrees F pre-heated oven for 10 minutes. While crust is baking, roll out remaining dough for the top and beat the egg white. Remove crust from oven and pour in boiling hot filling. Place dough on top, trim around edges, brush with egg white, cut several slits in top, and put back in oven for 20 minutes.

MERINGUE FOR PIE

Use standard meringue recipe or purchase a box of fluffy white frosting mix, making sure that it is fat free and made from egg whites. Prepare as per instructions and pile on top of your pie. Place in a preheated 500 degrees F oven for just a minute or so until browned to suit you. Note: For cold refrigerated pies you may use the whipped yogurt cream topping on page 316.

LEMON MERINGUE PIE

    Jell-O® brand lemon pie filling mix
    prepared with Egg Beaters® eggs substitute
1   package fluffy white frosting mix (fat free)
1   pie crust baked to light brown

    Prepare filling and spoon into pie shell. Top with frosting mix and place in preheated 500 degree oven for 1 minute to brown the meringue.

BANANA CREME PIE

1   package Jell-O® brand banana cream
    cook and serve pudding and pie filling
1   package fluffy white frosting mix (fat free)
1   large banana, sliced

    Prepare filling using non-fat milk, add banana and spoon into cool pie shell. Cover with fluffy white meringue and place in preheated 500 degree oven for one minute to brown meringue.

BOURBON PIE OR MOCK PECAN PIE
(made by omitting the bourbon)

    This is a very fine replacement for pecan pie. These pies come in about one-plus gram of fat per slice, whereas traditional pecan pie will average 32 grams of fat per slice. You would have to eat about 5 whole bourbon pies to equal just one slice of regular pecan pie. So, kick back and enjoy.

BOURBON PIE

1	buttermilk biscuit pie dough, uncooked, page 278
1	cup dark corn syrup
1	cup sugar
2	tablespoons Butter Buds® flavored granules
2	tablespoons bourbon whiskey
1	teaspoon vanilla
1/2	cup oatmeal, regular and uncooked
1/2	cup cooked rice
1/2	cup Egg Beaters® egg substitute

Except for rice and oats beat other ingredients for 2 or 3 minutes. Add rice and oats and mix. Pour into uncooked pie shell and in a 350 degrees preheated oven, bake for 60 minutes until center is set. There will be some liquid but filling will be firm.

NOTE: For mock pecan pie just omit the bourbon whiskey. You'll fool a lot of people

CRUSTLESS PUMPKIN PIE

1	16 oz can pumkin
1	can evaporated skimmed milk
3/4	cup Egg Beaters® egg substitute
3/4	cup sugar
1/2	cup flour
1 1/2	teaspoon pumpkin pie spice
3/4	teaspoon baking powder
1/8	teaspoon salt

1/2   cup regular rolled oats

Except for the oats, beat and thoroughly mix all ingredients. Fold in oats and spoon into a round deep casserole dish. This makes one big pie or two small ones. Bake in preheated 350 degree oven for 50 minutes or until toothpick or knife inserted in center comes out clean. Sprinkle powdered sugar on top and serve when cool.

APPLE OR CHERRY PIE

1   16 oz can pie filling (fat free)
1   pie shell, uncooked page 278
      or use 2 crust recipe page 280

Spoon pie filling into cooked pie shell. If desired use additional pie dough cut in strips to make a lattice top for the pie. Bake in preheated 375 degree oven for 25 minutes. to prevent over browning of crust, cover with aluminum foil.

KEY LIME PIE

1/4   cup water
1   envelope unflavored gelatin
1/2   cup fresh lime juice
        Grated rind of one lime
1   package fluffy white frosting mix (fat free)
1   cup evaporated skimmed milk
1   cup Egg Beaters® egg substitute
        Green food coloring
        9-inch chocolate cake crumb pie crust
        from page 279

Dissolve gelatin in 1/4 cup hot water, add milk, eggs, lime juice, and lime rind. Bring to simmer over medium heat, stirring constantly. Simmer for 2 or 3 minutes and remove from heat. Prepare frosting mix as per directions, adding one or two drops of food coloring while beating. Add one drop of food coloring to egg mixture, also. Gently fold frosting mix into egg mixture. Spoon out into pie crust and chill. Garnish with wafer thin slices of fresh lime prior to serving.

NO SUGAR SOUR CREAM APPLE RAISIN PIE

THE FILLING

1/2	cup water
3	cups sliced Granny Smith apples
1	cup apple juice concentrate
1	tablespoon cornstarch
1	teaspoon apple pie spice
1	cup sour cream from page
	Artificial sweetener to taste
	Two-crust pie crust from page 280

In a sauce pan, bring apples and water to a boil and simmer for 5 minutes. Meanwhile, combine in a bowl the apple juice concentrate, cornstarch, and apple pie spice. Then pour into the apples and simmer for another 5 minutes. Remove from heat and fold in sour cream. Add artificial sweetener, if desired. Pour into pie crust and follow pie crust directions.

SOUR CREAM APPLE PIE

6	medium apples, peeled, cored and sliced thin
2/3	cup brown sugar
1/4	teaspoon cinnamon

1/8   teaspoon nutmeg
1/8   teaspoon salt
1   tablespoon cornstarch
1   cup sour cream from page 321
1   egg white, lighlty beaten

Preheat oven to 400 degrees F. In mixing bowl combine everything but the sour cream. Make sure apples are well coated. Place in biscuit pie crust from page 278. Pour sour cream over top of apples, fold over pie crust then brush pie crust wih egg white and dust with sugar and/or cinnamon if desired.

CINNAMON PEACH PIE

1   29 oz can sliced peaches in heavy syrup
1   teaspoon cinnamon
2   tablespoons corn starch

Mix ingredients in sauce pan and bring to a boil, being careful not to burn. Pour out into biscuit pie crust from page 278 and fold excess pie crust over to center of pie and sprinkle crust with sugar and cinnamon. Bake in a preheated 400 degree oven for 10 minutes. Reduce temperature to 350 degrees and continue baking for 20 minutes more. Remove pie from oven and allow to cool.

BASIC COBBLER BATTER

This batter can be spooned into all sorts of combinations to make delicious cobblers.

2   cups flour
3   teaspoons baking powder
1   tablespoon sugar (omit for veggie cobblers)

1/2   cup non-fat milk powder
       Water and fruit juice or nectar as needed

Mix dry ingredients together, then add liquid to make a spoonable batter. Note: For vegetable cobblers, omit sugar and fruit juice.

COBBLERS

When making these fruit cobblers, a basic rule to follow is that for every 16 oz can of fruit (about 2 cups) or equivalent fresh fruit and juice, add 1 1/2 tablespoon of cornstarch. This will thicken your cobbler juice to a nice consistency. Also, add sugar to suit your tastes if using fresh tart fruit. Fill baking dish only 1/2 full, as dough will rise.

PEACH AND RASPBERRY COBBLER

2   cups sliced canned peaches in heavy syrup
2   cups frozen raspberries with sugar added
     to taste
3   tablespoons corn starch

Combine ingredients and spoon one half into baking dish. Spoon cobbler batter from page onto fruit. Cover batter with remaining fruit and bake in 350 degree preheated oven for about 45 minutes until toothpick stuck into dough comes out clean.

BLACKBERRY COBBLER

4   cups canned blackberries and juice sweetened
     to taste
3   tablespoons corn starch
     Cobbler batter from page 285

Combine berries and corn starch and spoon one half into baking dish. Spoon batter onto fruit. Pour remaining berries on top of batter and bake in preheated 350 degree oven for 45 minutes or until toothpick stuck in batter dough comes out clean.

FRESH STRAWBERRY COBBLER

1   Pint fresh strawberries, sliced,
         sweetened to taste
1   cup cranberry-raspberry juice
1 1/2   tablespoons cornstarch
         Cobbler batter from page 285

Combine fruit, juice, and cornstarch, spoon one half into baking dish. Spoon batter onto fruit. Spoon rest of fruit on top of batter. Bake in preheated 350 degree oven for 45 minutes or until a toothpick stuck into dough comes out clean.

PUDDINGS

Pudding mixes are fine to use as long as they contain no fat. Just use non-fat ingredients in preparing the mix. That is, use Egg Beaters® if eggs are called for and non-fat milk if milk is called for. Your puddings should be very near fat free.

BANANA ANGEL PUDDING

2   cups angel food cake broken into small
         bite-size pieces
1   box vanilla pudding cooked with
         non-fat milk
1   sliced large banana

Mix ingredients and chill.

RICE PUDDING

2	cups water
1	cup raisins
2	cups instant rice
2	tablespoons sugar
1/2	cup non-fat frozen yogurt

Bring water, raisins, and sugar to a boil. Add rice and remove from heat. After 5 minutes, add frozen yogurt to rice. Spoon into a casserole dish and bake at 400 degrees for 30 minutes.

WHISKEY BREAD PUDDING

1	cup Egg Beaters® egg substitute
2	cups non-fat milk
1/4	cup sugar
1/2	oz your favorite whiskey
1/2	teaspoon cinnamon
1/2	teaspoon cinnamon
1/2	teaspoon vanilla
1/8	teaspoon salt
2 1/2	cups dry non-fat bread cubes
1/3	cup raisins

In mixing bowl, beat Egg Beaters®, milk, sugar, whiskey, cinnamon, vanilla, and salt. Place bread in baking dish, sprinkle raisins on top, and pour egg mixture over all. Bake in preheated 350 degree oven for 30 to 40 minutes until toothpick inserted in center comes out clean.

BAKED CUSTARD CRUSTS

2 or 3	slices of homemade bread (Irish soda bread from page 269 or salt-risin' pumpkin bread from page 257 are just excellent breads for this recipe)
1	can evaporated skim milk
1/4	cup sugar
2	egg whites, slightly beaten
1/4	teaspoon nutmeg
	syrup (maple is great)

Preheat oven to 400 degrees F. Beat egg whites for 2 or 3 minutes, add milk and nutmeg. Place bread slices in a pie dish or pan and pour milk/egg mixture on top. Turn bread over to coat, then place in oven for 20 minutes. Remove and serve hot, topped with a splash of syrup.

BOURBON BREAD PUDDING

	Crusty bread
1/2	cup raisins
1	can evaporated skim milk
2	egg whites, slightly beaten
1/4	cup sugar
1/4	teaspoon nutmeg
1	oz bourbon

Preheat oven to 350 degrees F. Slice bread, preferable homemade, 1/2- to 3/4-inch thick and place in the bottom of an ovenproof pie dish or pan. Mix raisins in with bread. Beat egg white for a minute or so, add sugar, milk, and bourbon, mix thoroughly, and pour over bread. Sprinkle with nutmeg and bake for 30 minutes.

When serving, splash on a bit of maple syrup, and enjoy.

*Note: For lemon bread pudding, replace bourbon with grated rind of 1/2 lemon and juice from 1/2 lemon.

*For rum pudding, replace bourbon with 2 teaspoons rum flavoring.

*For vanilla pudding, replace bourbon with 1 teaspoon vanilla extract.

CAKES AND FROSTINGS

Most cakes today are loaded with fat, within the cake itself, the frosting, or both. However, it wasn't always this way. Eggs (with their fat yolks) were not readily available to city folks, in days gone by, and believe it or not - animal fat was also in short supply. Consequently, the celebratory cakes were often crafted without the use of eggs or fat.

OLDE, OLDE FASHIONED CAKE
Circa 1710

In 1835, when great-great grandfather Zebulon Rose and his wife Sarah pulled up stakes and left Boston Town, it was an event filled with fear and great apprehensions. A trip like that today can be made in a day, while it took them, literally years. You see, they were headed west to the Kentucky territory.

Neatly tucked into the hand-made, dove-tailed recipe box, among other things, were Sarah's notes on how to make a simple brown sugar-raisin cake. The recipe hadn't always contained brown sugar and raisins. In fact, it had been passed down to her as an old English recipe that used wild honey for a sweetener and dried local berries instead of the Mediterranean raisins (sometimes called currants) she was used to. Wild honey in Boston Town was rare, whereas brown sugar from the West Indies was plentiful. In Kentucky, the recipe would revert back to the use of wild honey and prunes made from an abundant supply of wild plums.

The leavening agent also changed from brewers yeast to what we now call baking powder.

What has remained constant is the dutch oven to cook it in, the whole grain flour, skimmed milk, and the apple butter used in the self-contained icing.

This is a robust, rich, moist cake in the old world country tradition, vastly different from present day "air" cake. The consumption of this cake carries with it an obligatory requirement, which is: as you sit down with your cake in front of you, fork in hand, pause for just a moment and imagine how your ancestors of 1835 would have received this special treat.

Enjoy!

THE CAKE

4	egg whites, beaten stiff
2 1/4	cups whole wheat flour
1 1/2	cups brown sugar
3	teaspoons baking powder
1	teaspoon salt
1	cup raisins
1	cup cooked and drained whole grain barley or wheat berries
1	cup skimmed milk

THE ICING

1	cup brown sugar

1   cup apple butter
Preheat oven to 375 degrees. In 10-inch dutch oven or 10-inch deep cake pan spread evenly on bottom, one cup brown sugar. Using a teaspoon, spoon 1 cup apple butter on top of brown sugar. Set aside. Beat egg whites stiff and set aside. In mixing bowl combine and mix thoroughly: 2 1/4 cups whole wheat flour, 1 1/2 cups brown sugar, 3 teaspoons baking powder, 1 teaspoon salt. Add to mixing bowl and mix well: 1 cup raisins, 1 cup cooked and drained whole grain barley or wheat berries, 1 cup skimmed milk. Fold in egg whites and pour mixture into dutch oven on top of brown sugar and apple butter.

Bake for 50 minutes or until inserted toothpick comes out clean. Remove from oven, run a knife around cake to loosen, place a plate on top of the cake and turn upside down thereby removing cake from dutch oven. In the bottom of the dutch oven is your icing for this cake. Spoon icing onto cake and serve hot or cold with a cup of hot fresh coffee.

LEMON ANGEL CAKE

1   angel food cake already cooked
1   package Jell-O® lemon pudding mix
(not instant)
Thin lemon slices
Fresh mint sprigs

Prepare pudding using Egg Beaters® egg substitute instead of regular eggs. Place cake on large cake dish and cover with lemon pudding. Garnish around base of cake with lemon slices and mint sprigs alternating. This is an elegant, yet quite simple dessert.

FAT-FREE CHOCOLATE CAKE

1 1/4   cups flour
1   cup sugar
1/2   cup unsweetened cocoa
1/4   cup cornstarch
1/2   teaspoon baking soda
1/2   teaspoon salt
1/2   cup Egg Beaters® egg substitute
1   cup water
1/2   cup corn syrup

In large bowl combine dry ingredients. Mix well. In smaller bowl, mix eggs, water, and corn syrup. Stir into dry ingredients until smooth. Pour into non-stick Teflon cake pan. Bake 30 minutes in preheated 350 degree oven, or until toothpick test is passed. Remove to wire rack and cool thoroughly before icing. Ice with fluffy white frosting mix or creole mocha frosting from page 313.

BLACK WALNUT
CREAM CAKE OR TRIFLE

In the wonderful world of no-fat fare all nuts are an absolute no-no. However, the cravings sometimes surface and cry to be placated. Such as it was with black walnut cake like Mom use to make in the old wood cook stove. Black walnuts weighing in at 64 grams of fat per 4 ounces represents nearly 5 times the daily fat requirement for an average person. So real black walnuts were eliminated from all consideration, immediately. However, thanks to modern technology, you can obtain all the flavor and texture of black walnuts and yet do it fat-free. You'll need to take a trip to a local health food or specialty store and pick up some TVP® (Textured Vegetable Protein), and from your local grocer pick up a bottle of imitation black walnut extract. Place 1/4 cup of TVP® into a cup or glass and pour 1 tablespoon of walnut extract on top. Mix well, cover, and set aside for at least an hour. Now you have the flavor and texture to make a wonderful cream filled black walnut cake or black walnut raspberry cream trifle without the fat.

BLACK WALNUT CAKE

1	tablespoon imitation black walnut extract
1/4	cup TVP® mixed with imitation black walnut extract and allowed to sit for at least one hour
1 1/2	cups sugar
1/2	cup cold water
2	tablespoons baking powder
1/8	teaspoon salt
1	teaspoon vanilla extract
3/4	cup Egg Beaters® egg substitute
1 1/2	cups flour

In mixing bowl, beat Egg Beaters® for 3 or 4 minutes. Mix in water, sugar, baking powder, salt, and vanilla. Mix thoroughly but do not beat. Mix in flour to smooth consistency, then mix in TVP®. (Note: Reserve a small portion of flavored TVP® to sprinkle on top of the finished cake.) Pour into two 8-inch sure-release cake pans and bake in 350 degree preheated oven for 20 minutes or until toothpick placed in center of cake comes out clean.

THE FILLING - VANILLA, BUTTER, AND NUT CREAM

2/3   cup dry powdered non-fat milk
       Water to make 2 cups milk liquid
1   tablespoon Butter Buds® butter
       flavor granules
1/4   cup Egg Beaters® egg substitute
1/2   cup sugar
2   tablespoons cornstarch
1   teaspoon vanilla, butter, and nut extract

Mix ingredients in sauce pan and bring to boil on medium heat, stirring constantly. Remove from heat and allow to cool. Spread between layers of cake.

THE ICING

1 package fluffy white frosting (no fat) or use your own beaten egg white and sugar frosting recipe. Prepare as per instructions.

THE MECHANICS

Your cake pans should be the type that has a rotating removal device that extends from the center of your cake pans to the outside. If you don't have this type of pan and your cake won't come free except in pieces, then proceed on to the "Contingency Trifle". Wax paper lined cake pans work well, as do spring form cake pans. Assuming your cake, does come out intact, place one layer in a regular plate so that the rounded top is on the bottom. Insert a tablespoon into this layer and twirl, making openings so that the filling can seep down into the bottom layer. Ten or twelve such openings should be enough. Spoon on cooled filling and spread. Place top layer on filling and hold in place by inserting four or five toothpicks through both layers. Spoon on fluffy white frosting and sprinkle with leftover TVP®.

THE CONTINGENCY - BLACK WALNUT-RASPBERRY TRIFLE

If your cake comes out in pieces, or if you just want to make a trifle, then assemble six tall, narrow glasses (Parfait, ice cream soda, or Tom Collins glasses will work) and one package of frozen whole unsweetened raspberries, next fold fluffy white icing into filling. Spoon into each glass alternating layers of filling/icing mixture, cake pieces (bite size), and raspberries. Make sure filling/icing ends up topping your trifle. Sprinkle on TVP®, garnish with a sprig of mint, and enjoy - fat free!

PINEAPPLE MAYONNAISE CAKE WITH CREAM FILLING

2 1/4   cups all-purpose flour
1   cup sugar
1   teaspoon baking powder
2   teaspoons baking soda
1   cup cold water
1   teaspoon vanilla
1   cup fat-free mayonnaise
2   cups pineapple, crushed and drained
1   teaspoon imitation butter flavoring
        Vegetable spray

Preheat oven to 350 degrees F. In a large mixing bowl, combine and mix thoroughly the flour, sugar, baking powder, and baking soda. In another bowl, combine and mix thoroughly the water, vanilla, mayonnaise, pineapple, and butter flavoring. Combine the two bowls and mix well - QUICKLY! Pour into a 10-inch spring form pan and bake for 50 minutes or until toothpick inserted into cake comes out clean. Remove, cool, and split into 2 layers. Onto the first layer, spoon the following filling. Place the remaining layer on top and use several tooth picks to hold the layers together. Then ice with fluffy white frosting mix.

PINEAPPLE FILLING

1	can, 5 1/2 oz crushed pineapple with juice
1	teaspoon imitation butter flavor
1	cup water
1/3	cup non-fat milk powder
1/4	cup Egg Beaters® egg substitute
1/2	cup sugar
2	tablespoons corn starch

Mix ingredients in large sauce pan and bring to a boil. Remove from heat, allow to cool somewhat, and use for cake filling.

PINEAPPLE RUM CAKE

1 1/4	cups flour
1	cup sugar
1/4	cup cornstarch
1/2	teaspoon baking soda
1/2	teaspoon salt
1/2	cup Egg Beaters® egg beaters
1/4	cup pineapple juice from can of pineapple
3/4	cup water

1/2	cup corn syrup
1	cup pineapple chunks
1	cup dark brown sugar
2	teaspoons rum flavoring

Preheat oven to 350 degrees F. Except for dark brown sugar, combine all ingredients, do not beat. Place dark brown sugar in bottom of 9-inch spring-form cake pan. Spoon cake mixture on top and bake for 45 minutes or until toothpick in center comes out clean. Remove and cool.

PINEAPPLE UP-SIDE-DOWN CAKE

1	cup Egg Beaters® egg substitute
1 1/2	cups sugar
2 1/4	cup flour
3	teaspoons baking powder
1	teaspoon salt
1	cup non-fat liquid milk

1 1/2	teaspoon vanilla
1 20	oz. can pineapple slices
	Maraschino cherries
1	cup dark brown sugar

Preheat oven to 350 degrees F. In mixing bowl, beat Egg Beaters® for 3 or 4 minutes until frothy and add vanilla. In bottom of 10-inch spring form cake pan, spread dark brown sugar and space pineapple slices uniformly with cherries in centers of each slice. In separate mixing bowl, mix rest of ingredients thoroughly. Fold in eggs and mix well. Pour into cake pan on top of pineapple. Bake for 50 minutes or until toothpick in center of cake comes out clean.

DARK SWEET CHERRY UP-SIDE-DOWN CAKE

Use previous pineapple up-side-down cake recipe, substituting a 17-ounce can of dark, sweet, pitted cherries for the pineapple.

CINNAMON-PEACH UP-SIDE-DOWN CAKE

Using previous pineapple up-side-down cake recipe, substituting a 17- to 20- ounce can of sliced peaches for the pineapple. Sprinkle 1 teaspoon of cinnamon on top of the peaches.

CRANBERRY-RAISIN CAKE

1 1/2	cups flour
1/8	teaspoon salt
2	teaspoons baking soda
1	cup sugar
1/2	cup cold water
1	teaspoon vanilla
1	cup canned whole cranberries
1/2	cup raisins
	Vegetable spray

Preheat oven to 350 degrees F. In a large mixing bowl, combine and mix thoroughly the flour, salt, soda, and sugar. In a separate bowl, combine and mix thoroughly the water, vanilla, cranberries, and raisins. Combine the two bowls and mix - QUICKLY! Pour into a 9- or 10-inch spring form pan that has been veggie-sprayed and flour dusted. Bake for 45 minutes or until toothpick inserted in cake comes out clean.

APPLE BUTTER RAISIN CAKE

1 1/4   cup self-rising flour
1   cup dark sugar
1/4   cup corn starch
1   teaspoon imitation butter flavoring
1/2   teaspoon vanilla extract
1/2   cup Egg Beaters® egg substitute
1 1/4   cup apple butter
1/2   cup dark corn syrup
1/2   cup raisins
         Vegetable spray

Preheat oven to 350 degrees F. In a large mixing bowl, combine and mix thoroughly the flour, sugar, and corn starch. In another bowl, beat eggs for 3 to 4 minutes, then add butter flavoring, vanilla, apple butter, corn syrup, and raisins, mixing well. Combine the two bowls, mix thoroughly but quickly, and pour into a 9- or 10-inch spring form, veggie-sprayed cake pan. Bake for 40 to 45 minutes until toothpick inserted in center of cake comes out clean.

COCONUT CAKE

1 1/2   cup self-rising flour
1   cup sugar
1/4   cup cornstarch
1/2   cup Egg Beaters® egg substitute
1   teaspoon imitation butter flavor
1   cup cold water
1/2   cup corn syrup
1   tablespoon imitation coconut extract
         Vegetable spray

Preheat oven to 350 degrees F. In a large mixing bowl, combine and mix thoroughly the flour, sugar, and corn starch. In another bowl, beat eggs for 3 or 4 minutes. Add and mix the butter flavor, water, corn syrup, and coconut flavoring. Combine the two bowls, mix thoroughly but quickly, and pour into a veggie-sprayed 9- or 10-inch spring form cake pan. Bake for 40- to 45 minutes or until toothpick inserted in center of cake comes out clean.

BOURBON CARROT CAKE

2   cups all-purpose flour
1 1/2 cups granulated sugar
1   teaspoon baking soda
1   teaspoon baking powder
1   teaspoon cinnamon
1/2   cup whole raisins
1   oz bourbon (optional)
3/4   cup pureed raisins in 1/2 cup cold water
1   cup Egg Beaters® egg substitute
3   cups shredded carrots

Preheat oven to 325 degrees F. Combine flour, sugar, soda, baking powder, cinnamon and mix well. In a blender or food processor, puree raisins with water and bourbon. Combine all ingredients and mix until moist. Beat at medium speed for two minutes. Pour into a 12 x 9 x 2 inch greased and floured baking pan. Bake for 50 minutes until toothpick inserted comes out clean. If possible, allow this cake to sit around for a day or so. It ages very well. As an option, consider sprinkling cake with liqueur syrup from page 316 prior to aging. Frost cake with fluffy yogurt frosting from page 313 and serve.

STRAWBERRY SHORTCAKE

SHORTCAKE BATTER

	Sour Cream biscuit dough from page 266
1/4	cup sugar
2	teaspoons imitation butter flavoring
1	teaspoon vanilla flavoring
1/4	cup water (to make consistency of cake batter)

FRUIT FILLING

4	cups fresh sliced strawberries
1/2	cup strawberry glaze
	Sugar or sweetener to taste
	Whipped yogurt cream topping from page 316

Preheat oven to 375 degrees F. To biscuit dough, add 1/4 cup sugar, butter flavoring, and vanilla flavoring. Mix well to consistency of cake batter. Bake in veggie-sprayed 9-inch cake pan (spring form works best) for 45 minutes. Remove and cool. Split cake into 2 layers using a good knife. Invert rounded top layer of cake and place on a plate. Combine strawberries, glaze, and sweetener and spoon 1/2 onto bottom layer. Place other layer on top of strawberries, secure with several toothpicks, then spoon on remaining strawberries. Prepare whipped yogurt cream topping and spoon generously and decoratively onto top of cake. Chill and serve. Note: Just change the selection of fruit for other delicious shortcakes for instance use fresh raspberries in season or pineapple anytime.

WHIPPED CREAM CAKE

3   egg whites
3/4   cup nonfat yogurt
1/2   cup nonfat milk powder
1/2   cup cold water
1   teaspoon almond flavoring
2   cups self-rising flour
1 1/2 cups sugar

Preheat oven to 325 degrees F. Beat egg whites until stiff and set aside. Combine yogurt and milk powder and beat until stiff then gently fold into egg whites. Gradually fold in the cold water and almond flavoring. Fold flour and sugar into creamy mixture. Pour into two 8 inch layer pans lined in the bottom with wax paper. Top one layer with bake-on icing from page 315. Bake for 35 minutes until done. Remove and cool. Use your favorite filling in between layers or use fresh fruit or jam or a mixture of tthe two, or just ice cake as desired.

Note: For a really simple and quick filling cover bottom layer with slices of pineapple and spoon on 4 or 5 tablespoons of pineapple juice or use peaches and peach juice or cherries and cherry juice or whatever you like.

CREAM CHEESE CHEESE CAKE

(LESS THAN 1/2 GRAM PER 1/16TH CAKE)

3   cups cream cheese from page 322
3/4   cup sugar
1/2   cup evaporated skim milk
8   egg whites

4	tablespoons flour
1	teaspoon vanilla flavoring
1	teaspoon lemon flavoring
1	teaspoon imitation butter flavoring
	Vegetable spray
	Cornflake crumbs

Preheat oven to 350 degrees F. Mix cheese, sugar, and milk in a large mixing bowl. In another mixing bowl, lightly beat egg whites and mix in flour, vanilla, butter, and lemon flavoring. Make sure flour is evenly blended, then combine the two bowls. Mix and pour into a veggie-sprayed, cornflake crumb dusted, 9-inch, spring form cake pan. Place cake pan in a sheet pan containing about 1/2-inch water and place in oven. After 10 minutes, reduce heat to 200 degrees F. Bake for two hours. Turn off heat and slightly open the oven door and allow cake to sit in oven for one more hour. Remove and chill for at least 2 hours (preferably overnight) before serving. Note: Make a special effort NOT to beat a lot of air into the batter. Note: After cooling, cake may be topped with fresh strawberry, pineapple chunks, blue berries, or cherries along with the appropriate glaze.

CHOCOLATE FUDGE CHEESECAKE
(1.5 GRAMS OF FAT PER 1/16TH CAKE)

1	box "lite" brownie mix (1 gram fat per serving
2	cups fat free cottage cheese, drained
2	cups cream cheese from page 322
1	cup sugar
8	egg whites
2/3	cup evaporated skim milk
4	tablespoons flour

1	teaspoon vanilla flavoring
1	teaspoon butter flavoring
1	teaspoon lemon flavoring
	Vegetable spray
	Corn flake crumbs

Preheat oven to 350 degrees F. Prepare brownie mix as per directions. Pour 1/2 of the mix into a 9-inch spring form cake pan that has been veggie sprayed and dusted with corn flake crumbs. Bake for 20 minutes. To remaining batter, add 1/2 cup raisins and mix well. Spoon onto veggie-sprayed cookie sheet one tablespoon at a time for some scrumptious chocolate raisin cookies. Bake cookies with other cake and remove at the same time. While brownie mix is cooking, prepare in a large mixing bowl the cream cheese, milk, and sugar. Cream them together - don't beat them! In another mixing bowl force cottage cheese through sieve or strainer to reduce the size of curd. Add egg whites, vanilla, lemon juice, lenom rind, butter flavoring, and flour. Mix well. If using a mixer, do not beat a lot of air into mixture. Combine two bowls and pour on top of cooked brownie mix. Bake at 350 degrees F for 10 minutes, reduce heat to 200 degrees F and cook for 2 hours. Turn heat off, slightly oven for one hour. Chill in refrigerator overnight. Note: For regular cheese cake, omit the chocolate brownie mix.

Note: Fat content for regular non-fat cheesecake (less brownie mix) is approximately .75 grams per 1/16th cake.

MY FAVORITE BROWNIES

1   package "lite" brownie mix
      (1 gram per serving)
1   cup raisins
1/4   cup "walnuts" from page 322 (optional)

To brownie mix add raisins and "walnuts" and follow mix directions.

TRIFLES

A beautiful outrageous fat-free dessert.

Fruit, sweetened to taste
Heavy dessert cream from page 316
Cake, left-over, even a little stale is okay

In tall glass, pour a little heavy cream in the bottom, then add alternate layers of fruit and cake to fill. Top off with more heavy cream and garnish with a maraschino cherry and a sprig of fresh mint.

CREPES

These are french pancakes. They should be thin, yet fluffy - not gummy and chewy. Wrap them around your favorite sweetened fruit, sprinkle on some powdered sugar, top with a spoon of sweetened sour cream or heavy dessert cream page   and you have a definite winner.

CREPE BATTER

1   cup Krusteaz® brand oat bran
      lite complete pancake mix

1   cup Egg Beaters® egg substitute
     Water to make batter the consistency
     of heavy cream

Veggie spray a medium hot griddle or heavy skillet. Spoon on batter and brown on both sides. Fry a quantity, then assemble crepes. these crepes also go well with meat, seafood, and vegetable fillings.

SPECIALTY DESSERTS

These desserts work well in a long-stemmed margarita glass. The possible combinations are endless, so let your imagination rule the day.

    Non-fat cake
    Non-fat dairy frozen dessert
    Fruit, sweetened to taste or pureed fruit
    or sauce

Place a small scoop of frozen dessert in bottom of glass. Place slice or small squares of cake on top. Spoon fruit or sauce or pureed fruit onto cake. Place another small scoop of frozen dessert beside cake. Garnish with spring of fresh mint or some fruit.

Another specialty dessert full of surprises is Baked Alaska.

INDIVIDUAL BAKED ALASKA

    Fat free pound cake
    Fat free frozen dessert
    Fluffy white frosting mix (fat free),

Prepare frosting as per directions.

On baking sheet, arrange flat separated slices of pound cake. Top with a scoop of fat-free ice cream or other frozen dessert. Spoon on frosting mix to cover ice cream and cake. Place in preheated 500 degree oven for 3 minutes until brown. Serve immediately. Note: Spoon fresh or frozen raspberries onto cake before ice cream for a wonderful variation.

COOKIES

The availability and variety of fat-free cookies and frozen desserts is rapidly increasing. Just be sure to purchase products "fat-free" or "non-fat".

CHOCOLATE COVERED CHERRY COOKIES

MAKES 20 COOKIES - 1/2 GRAM OF FAT PER COOKIE

1/3	package "light" brownie mix (1 gram of fat per serving) with
1/3	required water
20	maraschino cherries, drained

Preheat oven to 375 degrees F. Dry cherries on a paper towel. Mix 1/3 brownie mix with 1/3 the required water. Add cherries and mix until covered with brownie mix. On veggie-sprayed cookie sheet, spoon cherries with approximately 1 tablespoon of brownie mix per cherry. Allow room for cookie to spread. Bake for 10 minutes. Allow to cool.

CHOCOLATE RAISIN COOKIES

MAKES 20 COOKIES - 1/2 GRAM OF FAT PER COOKIE

1/3	package "lite" brownie mix (1 gram of fat per serving)
1/3	water as required per Brownie mix directions
3/4	cup raisins Vegetable spray

Preheat oven to 375 degrees F. Mix brownie mix according to directions. Add raisins and spoon onto veggie-sprayed cookie sheet in about 1 tablespoon portions. Bake for 10 minutes. Remove and cool.

BROWN SUGAR RAISIN COOKIES

2 1/4	cups whole wheat flour
1 1/2	cups light brown sugar
3	teaspoons baking powder
1	teaspoon salt
1	cup raisins
1	cup whole grain barley, cooked and drained
1	cup non-fat skimmed milk

Combine and mix thoroughly the flour, sugar, baking powder, and salt. Add raisins, barley, and milk. Spoon onto cookie sheet and bake in a preheated 375 degree F oven for 8 to 10 minutes until done.

CHEWY CHOCOLATE COOKIES

MAKES TWO DOZEN

1 1/2   cup self-rising flour

1/2   cup sugar
1/2   cup cocoa powder
1/2   cup light or dark corn syrup
3   egg whites
       Vegetable spray

Preheat oven to 350 degrees F. In large mixing bowl, combine flour, sugar, and cocoa. Stir in corn syrup and egg whites until blended. Drop full teaspoons onto cookie sheet and bake for about 8 minutes until firm yet soft. Do not overbake. Remove and cool.

BROWNIE OATMEAL COOKIES
MAKES TWO DOZEN

2/3   cup self-rising flour
2/3   cup sugar
1   cup uncooked oatmeal
1/3   cup cocoa powder
2   egg whites
1/3   cup corn syrup (light or dark)
1   teaspoon vanilla
       Vegetable spray

Preheat oven to 350 degrees F. In large mixing bowl, combine flour, sugar, oatmeal, and cocoa powder. Add syrup, egg whites, and vanilla. Stir until everything is just moistened. Drop full teaspoons onto a veggie-sprayed cookie sheet. Bake for 8 minutes or until cookies are just set. Remove and cool.

OLD FASHION SUGAR COOKIES

1   cup lite white or yellow cake mix
1   cup self rising flour
1/3   cup sugar

1   egg white
1/2   teaspoon vanilla
1   teaspoon lemon juice
1/4   cup skimmed milk
         Vegetable spray

Combine and mix cake mix, flour and sugar. In another bowl, briefly whisk egg white, vanilla, lemon juice and skimmed milk. Combine liquid mixture with flour mixture, mix and form into ball and chill in refrigerator for at least one hour.
Preheat oven to 375 degrees.
Roll out dough to about 1/4 inch on lightly floured board or pastry cloth. Sprinkle with granulated sugar and cut into cookies. Bake on veggie sprayed sheet for 10 minutes.

VARIETIES OF SUGAR COOKIE

Sugar-Raisin Cookings - Add 1/2 cup raisins when mixing dough.

Sugar Cherry Cookies - Add 1/2 cup chopped glazed cherries when mixing dough.

Sugar Cinnamon Tarts - Roll out dough, cut with 2 inch cutter, brush with lightly beaten egg white and sprinkle with sugar and cinnamon (2 tablespoons sugar and 1/4 teaspoon cinnamon)

Sugar & Spice Cookies - Substitute brown for granulated sugar, omit vanilla and add 1/4 teaspoon cinnamon, 1/8 teaspoon cloves and 1/8 teaspoon nutmeg.

Sugar Raisin Spice - Add 1/2 cup raisins to spice cookies above.

Lemon-Sugar - Omit vanilla and add 1 teaspoon grated lemon rind and 1/2 teaspoon lemon flavoring.

Maple Pecan - Omit vanilla and add 1 teaspoon imitation vanilla butter and nut flavor, 1 tablespoon TVP®, and 1/4 teaspoon maple extract.

FRUIT STREUSEL MUFFINS

(MAKES 12 MUFFINS)

1 1/2	cups self-rising flour
3/4	cup sugar
1	tablespoon oat bran (optional)
2/3	cup yogurt, plain, non-fat
2/3	cup evaporated skim milk
1/2	cup crushed pineapple, blueberries, apples, etc.
	Vegetable spray

Streusel filling

1/3	cup sugar
1/2	teaspoon cinnamon

Preheat oven to 375 degrees F. In mixing bowl, combine, flour, yogurt, milk, and fruit. Fill veggie sprayed muffin tin 1/2 full. Place 1 teaspoon of filling on top, then add more batter to fill muffin tins 3/4 full. Bake for 30 minutes until browned. Serve warm.

PINEAPPLE FRITTERS

MAKES 12 MUFFINS

2	cups self-rising flour
1/4	cup sugar
1/2	cup crushed pineapple with some juice
2/3	cup non-fat yogurt
	Vegetable spray
	Powdered sugar

Preheat oven to 400 degrees F. Mix flour and sugar in mixing bowl. Quickly add pineapple and yogurt and stir. Spoon into veggie-sprayed muffin tin and pop into oven as quickly as possible. Bake for 30 minutes or until well browned. Remove and dust generously top and bottom and all parts in between with powdered sugar. Serve warm.

FLUFFY YOGURT FROSTING

1	package fluffy white frosting mix (no fat)
1/2	cup plus 1 tablespoon non-fat yogurt
2	teaspoons imitation butter flavoring

Prepare frosting mix as per directions, except use 1/2 cup nonfat yogurt for the 1/2 cup water that is called for. When thick and stiff, add butter flavoring and then spread on cooled cake. Note: Yogurt when boiled will separate and look yuckey. Not to worry, the small curds will give texture to your icing.

CREOLE MOCHA FROSTING

2	cups powdered sugar
4	tablespoons cocoa
2	teaspoons instant coffee powder

4   tablespoons boiling water
1   teaspoon vanilla
1   teaspoon hot water

Mix sugar and cocoa, add instant coffee dissolved in boiling water and vanilla. Stir until smooth. Add some additional hot water to make a smooth, manageable frosting.

SUGAR-FREE LEMON CREAM FROSTING

1/2   cup non-fat powdered milk powder
3/4   cup non-fat yogurt
2   tablespoons lemon juice
       Artificial sweetener equal to 1/2 cup sugar
       or to taste

Beat milk powder and yogurt until somewhat fluffy (about 3 minutes). Pour in the lemon juice and continue beating until stiff. Fold in sweetener until mixed. Note: Substitute other flavors for the lemon juice to insure variety.

Betty Crocker offers an excellent fat-free fluffy white frosting mix that goes well with almost any cake.

Use your favorite recipe for angel food cake or sponge cakes.

CHOCOLATE FROSTING

1/2   package light fudge brownie mix
       (1 gram of fat per serving)
       Water as called for
       Powdered sugar as needed

Mix 1/2 package brownie mix as directed. Add powdered sugar and mix until consistency of thick frosting. For a more chocolaty tase add chocolate extract.

SWEETENED CREAM CHEESE FROSTING

1   cup cream cheese from page 322
1   cup powdered sugar

Blend, softened to room temperature cream cheese and sugar until creamy smooth.

BAKE-ON FROSTING

2   egg whites
1/4 teaspoon salt
2   cups brown sugar

Add salt to egg whites and beat until stiff. Beat in brown sugar and set aside until cake batter is poured into cake pan then spoon this frosting on top of cake batter and bake cake for at least 35 minutes.

Note: Top of frosting may be lightly sprinkled with corn flake crumbs.

* For burnt orange frosting add 2 teaspoons orange flavoring.

* For coconut frosting add 1 teaspoon coconut flavoring.

LIQUEUR SYRUP FOR LAYER CAKES
MAKES ABOUT ONE CUP

3/4   cup hot water
1/4   cup sugar
4   tablespoons rum, orange liqueur,
       flavored brandies, or 1 tablespoon
       vanilla extract

Dissolve sugar in hot water, add flavoring and use by spooning or sprinkling onto layers of cake just prior to icing or onto shortcake just prior to the fruit.

WHIPPED YOGURT CREAM TOPPING

1/2   cup non-fat powdered milk powder
3/4   cup non-fat yogurt
2   tablespoons lemon juice
1/2   cup sugar

Beat milk powder and yogurt until somewhat fluffy (about 3 minutes). Pour in lemon juice and continue beating until stiff. Fold in sugar and serve as whip cream topping.

HEAVY DESSERT CREAM

This "cream" pours well on cobblers, cake, fruit, shortcake, or pies.

Fat-free vanilla frozen dessert
(Simple Pleasures® is excellent)

Set out desired amount in refrigerator to thaw out. This also works as a fat-free creamer in coffee.

WHIPPED CREAM

This recipe is accomplished quite well by simply reconstructing our cream minus the butterfat. Canned Evaporated skim milk is a sweet and tasty product. It does not have the twang associated with evaporated whole milk. The flavor of butterfat is obtained by using a liquid butter flavor. Since the basic recipe contains 1/2 cup of evaporated skim milk and 4/10th of 1 gram of fat, the entire bowlful of whipped cream will contain only 4/10ths of 1 gram of fat. A low sugar version can be created by using artificial sweetener in place of sugar. However, it doesn't stay whipped as long. This whipped cream is so low in fat that you can generously ladle it onto your dessert and no one gets fat, and it tastes outrageous.

BASIC WHIPPED CREAM DESSERT TOPPING

1	teaspoon unflavored gelatin dissolved in
3	tablespoons of boiling water, then cooled
1/2	cup evaporated skim milk, chilled
1/2	tablespoon sugar or one packet artificial sweetener
1/2	teaspoon liquid butter flavor

Combine and beat in a mixing bowl until cream holds its peak. Serve.

VARIATIONS OF WHIPPED CREAM

BUTTER RUM CREAM

Add 1/2 teaspoon rum flavor

BRANDIED CREAM

Add 1/2 teaspoon brandy flavor

LEMON CREAM

Add 1/2 teaspoon lemon flavor

COCONUT BUTTER CREAM

Add 1/2 teaspoon coconut flavor

MOCHA CREAM

Add 1/2 chocolate extract and 1/2 teaspoon instant coffee powder

SIMPLE WHIPPED CREAM TOPPING

3/4	cup cold evaporated skimmed milk
1/2	cup nonfat milk powder
1	teaspoon lemon juice
1	teaspoon imitation butter flavoring
1/2	cup sugar

Whip evaporated milk and milk powder until stiff; fold in lemon juice, butter flavoring and sugar. Serve cold.

REALLY QUICK HOT CHOCOLATE SAUCE

1/3	package "lite" brownie mix (1 gram per serving)
1/3	cup hot tap water

Combine brownie mix and water. If thinner sauce is desired, add a little more water. Serve hot over cake or ice cream.

CHEESECAKE CREAM TOPPING

1/2   cup hot water
1   teaspoon vanilla
1   teaspoon unflavored gelatin
1/4   cup sugar
1   cup sour cream made with evaporated
         skim milk from page 321

Dissolve gelatin in hot water, then add sugar and dissolve, pour into mixing bowl and add sour cream. Beat on high speed for 5 minutes. Chill and serve. Note: topping should be used fairly soon after beating as the gelatin tends to set up and it becomes firm.

XI. SPECIAL FOODS

FAT-FREE SOUR CREAM - CULTURED
MAKES TWO CUPS

1/2	cup water
12	oz can of evaporated non-fat milk
1	heaping teaspoon cultured "lite" sour cream (2 grams of fat per ounce or less)

Combine and mix thoroughly in a glass bowl or large drinking glass. Cover with plastic wrap and set aside at room temperature for 24 hours. After 24 hours, if you have used sour cream with a living culture, your mixture should have the consistency of a very heavy, thick cream. If you have used a blend or heat sterilized sour cream product containing a dead culture, then nothing will have happened and you'll have to find a different sour cream with a living culture. These cultures sometimes tend to grow in rope-like configurations and sometimes will appear stringy and goopy. Just stir briskly, thereby breaking down these strings. You now have essentially fat-free sour cream for use in most recipes.

The 12 oz can of evaporated non-fat milk contains about 1.2 grams of fat, and the sour cream used as a culture contains about 1 gram of fat. That totals 2.2 grams per 2 cups or 1.1 grams of fat per cup.

Note: Two cups of reconstituted non-fat powdered milk may be used instead of canned milk and water. This will result in an even lower fat content and an equally good sour cream product.

CREAM CHEESE

MAKES ABOUT EIGHT OUNCES OR ONE CUP

1   32 oz container of fat-free yogurt
Cheese cloth
Tall plastic container with a press-on top

In a bowl large enough to hold all of the yogurt, place cheese cloth at least 4 layers thick - allowing at least an extra 6 inches to lay over the side of the bowl. Spoon all of the yogurt into the cheese cloth, gather the cheese cloth around the top, and tie or twist at the top of the yogurt. Suspend yogurt inside plastic container at least 4 inches from the bottom so water may drain from yogurt. Allow to drain in refrigerator for at least 2 days. This cream cheese may be used in any recipe.

MOCK BLACK WALNUTS

1/4   cup TVP®
1   tablespoon black walnut flavoring extract

Combine, cover, and let sit for at least an hour. Use in recipes calling for black walnuts such as brownies.

Note: For almonds, use almond flavoring extract.

Note: TVP® (Textured Vegetable Protein) can be purchased at most health food stores or from Harvest Direct at 1-800-8-FLAVOR.

Appendix
Fat Content of Common Foods

ITEM ....GRAMS OF FAT

Almonds: whole, 1 ounce 15

Angel food cake: 1 piece .... trace

Apple: 1 apple .... trace

Apple juice: 1 cup .... trace

Applesauce: 1 cup .... trace

Apricots: 3 apricots .... trace

Apricot nectar: 1 cup .... trace

Artichoke: globe or french
1 artichoke .... trace

Asparagus: 4 spears .... trace

Avocado: california, whole, 1 avocado 30

Bacon: canadian, cooked, 2 slices 4

Bacon: cooked, 3 medium slices 9

Bagel: water, 3 1/2 inch diameter,
1 bagel 1

Baking powder: 1 teaspoon 0

Baking soda: 1 teaspoon 0

Banana: 1 banana 1

Barbecue sauce: 1 tablespoon .... trace

Beans: chick pea, garbanzos, 1 cup 4

Beans: Pork n' Beans, 1 cup 7

Beans: kidney, 1 cup 1

Beans: lentils, 1 cup 1

Beans: lima, 1 cup 1

Beans: pinto, 1 cup... 1

Beans: black eyed peas, 1 cup 1

Beans: green, 1 cup .... trace

Beans: white, navy, great northern,
1 cup 1

Beans: yellow, 1 cup................................. trace

Beef: dried, 2.5 ounces 4

Beef: ground patty, regular, broiled,
3 ounces 18

Beef: roast, relatively lean such as eye of
round, baked, lean only 2.6 ounces 5

Beef: steak, sirloin, broiled, lean only, 2.5
ounces 6

Beef: chuck blade, cooked, lean only,
3 ounces 13

Beer: 1 glass 0

Beets: 1 cup .... trace

Biscuit: from mix, 1 biscuit 3

Biscuit: from home recipe, 1 biscuit 5

Blackberries: raw, 1 cup 1

Bologna: 1 ounce slice. 2 slices 16

Bouillon cube: 1 teaspoon ...... trace to 1 gram
.... (check label)

Braunschweiger (liver sausage):
1 ounce per slice, 2 slices 18

Bread: Boston brown, 1 slice 1

Bread: cracked wheat, 1 slice 1

Bread: commercial French or
Italian with oil added, 1 slice 1

Bread: regular French or Italian no oil
added, 1 slice .... trace

Bread: mixed grain, 1 slice 1

Bread: Pita, 1 pita 1

Bread: wheat bread,enriched with oil
added, 1 piece 1

Bread: wheat bread, enriched,
no oil added, 1 piece .... trace

Bread: whole wheat, enriched oil added,
1 slice 1

Broccoli: cooked, 1 cup .... trace

Brussel Sprouts: cooked, 1 cup 1

Buffalo, 1 oz. lean, broiled .... less than 1

Butter: 1 tablespoon 11

Buttermilk: 1 cup 2

Cabbage: raw, 1 cup .... trace

Cake: angel food, 1 piece .... trace

Cake: coffee Cake, crumb, 1 piece 7

Cake: Devil's Food, 1 piece 8

Cake: carrot, with cream cheese frosting,
1 piece 21

Cake: yellow with chocolate frosting,
1 piece 8

Candy: caramels, plain or chocolate,
1 ounce 3

Candy: chocolate, milk, 1 ounce 9

Candy: gum drops .... trace

Candy: jelly beans, 1 ounce .... trace

Candy: marshmallows, 1 ounce 0
Candy: candy corn 0

Cantaloupe: 1/2 melon 1

Carbonated Beverage: all................................ 0

Carrot: raw, 1 cup..................................... trace

Cashew: dry roasted, 1 cup 63

Catfish: raw, 1 ounce 1

Cauliflower: raw, 1 cup.............................. trace

Celery: raw, 1 cup..................................... trace

Cereal: oatmeal, regular, 1 cup...................... 2

Cereal: corn flakes, 1 ounce .... trace

Cereal: 40% bran flakes, 1 ounce............ trace

Cereal: Grape-nuts, 1 ounce .... trace

Cereal: Raisin Bran, 1 ounce 1

Cereal: Frosted Flakes, 1 ounce .... trace

Cereal: Shredded Wheat, 1 ounce................ 1

Cereal: Wheat flakes.............................. trace

Cheese: blue, 1 ounce................................... 8

Cheese: cheddar, 1 ounce 9

Cheese: cottage, creamed, large curd,
1 cup 10

Cheese: cream, 1 ounce............................ 10

Cheese: feta, 1 ounce..............................6

Cheese: mozzarella, whole milk,
1 ounce...6

Cheese: mozzarella, part skim milk,
1 ounce...5

Cheese: muenster, 1 ounce...............9

Cheese: parmesan, 1 ounce 9

Cheese: provolone, 1 ounce 8

Cheese: ricotta, part skim, 1 cup 19

Cheese: swiss, 1 ounce.......................8

Cheese: processed american, 1 ounce 9

Cherries: sour, pitted, 1 cup .... trace

Chicken: fried with skin, batter dipped,
breast, 4.9 ounces 18

Chicken: fried flour coated, breast,
3.5 ounces 9 drumsticks, 1.7 ounces 7

Chicken: roasted, breast 3 ounces.................3
drumstick 1.6 ounces 2

Chicken: liver, cooked, 1 liver.......................1

Chick peas: (see beans)

Chocolate: baking, 1 ounce...........................15

Chocolate: pudding, with nonfat milk...........0

Clams: raw, meat only, 3 ounces 1

Cocoa: powder .... trace

Cocoa mix: with nonfat dry milk 1

Cookie: chocolate chip, 4 cookies 9

Cookie: fig bar, 4 cookies 4

Cookie: oatmeal with raisins, 4 cookies 10

Cookie: peanut butter, 4 cookies 14

Cookie: sandwich type, 4 cookies 8

Cookie: vanilla wafer, 10 cookies 7

Corn: chips, 1 ounce 9

Corn: sweet, 1 ear 1

Corn: canned, 1 cup 1

Corned beef: (see beef)

Corn starch: 1 tablespoon 0

Cottage cheese: (see cheese)

Crab: crab meat, canned, 1 cup 3

Crackers: cheese, 10 crackers 3

Crackers: graham, 2 crackers 3

Crackers: melba toast, 1 piece .... trace

Crackers: saltines, 4 crackers.......................... 1

Crackers: wheat, thin, 4 crackers................... 1

Cranberry juice: cocktail, 1 cup .... trace

Cranberry sauce: 1 cup............................ trace

Cream: half & half, 1 tablespoon 2

Cream: heavy, 1 tablespoon........................... 6

Cream: our dessert cream page 207 0

Cream: sour, 1 tablespoon............................. 3

Cream: extra light sour cream,
1 tablespoon 1

Creamer: dry, 1 teaspoon................................ 1

Cucumbers: 8 slices................................... trace

Dates: chopped, 1 cup 1

Dessert topping: whipped cream,
1 tablespoon 1

Doughnut: cake, 1 doughnut 12

Doughnut: yeast, 1 doughnut........................ 13

Duck: roasted, meat only, 1/2 duck............. 25

Egg: fresh, large, whole 1 egg 6

Egg: whites, large 0

Egg: yolks, large 6

Egg Substitute: Egg Beaters® 0

Eggplant: cooked, steamed, 1 cup 1

English muffin: 1 muffin 1

Fig: dried, 10 figs 2

Fish: (see flounder, sole, haddock,
herring, salmon, sardines, trout, tuna)

Fish sticks: 1 stick 3

Flounder: baked 1

Flour: white, 1 cup 1.5

Flour: whole wheat, 1 cup 2.5

Frankfurter: beef, cooked, 1 frank 13

Frankfurter: Hormel, Light & Lean®,
1 frank 1

Frosting mix: Betty Crocker®, fluffy
white, 1 package 0

Fruit cocktail: 1 cup .... trace

Garbanzos: (see beans)

Gelatin: flavored, 1 package .... trace

Gelatin: unflavored, 1 package .... trace

Gin: 1 ounce 0

Grapes: 10 grapes.............................. trace

Grapefruit: raw, 1/2 grapefruit................ trace

Grapefruit juice: raw, 1 cup..................... trace

Greens: spinach, mustard, 1 cup.............. trace

Haddock: raw, 1 ounce..............................0.1

Halibut: raw, 1 ounce 0.1

Ham: (see pork)

Hamburger: (see beef)

Herring: pickled, 3 ounces............................ 13

Honey: 1 cup 0

Honeydew: 1/10 melon............................ trace

Horseradish: 1 cup .... trace

Ice cream: regular, 1 cup............................ 14

Ice cream: frozen custard, 1 cup..................23

Ice cream: nonfat yogurt .... trace

Ice cream: Simple Pleasures®,
4 fluid ounces....................................less than 1

Ice milk: 1 cup 6

Jelly: 1 tablespoon.................................... trace

Lamb: chops, cooked, lean only,

1.7 ounces 7

Lamb: leg roasted, lean only, 2.6 ounces 6

Lard: 1 tablespoon 13

Lemon: 1 cup .... trace

Lemonade: 1 cup .... trace

Lentils: (see beans)

Lettuce: 1 head .... trace

Liquor: (see gin, bourbon, rum, vodka)

Liver: beef, 3 ounces 3.3

Lobster: 1 cup 2

Luncheon meat: spiced, canned,
2 slices 13

Luncheon meat: chopped ham, 2 slices 7

Luncheon meat: cooked ham, regular 6

Macaroni: elbow, enriched, 1 cup 1

Margarine: regular, 1 tablespoon 11

Margarine: soft 11

Margarine: diet lite 6

Milk: whole, 3.3% fat, 1 cup 8

Milk: 2 %, 1 cup 5

Milk: 1 %, 1 cup 3

Milk: canned, condensed, skim milk,
1 cup 1

Milk: canned, condensed, whole milk,
1 cup 19

Milk: dried, nonfat, 1 cup .... trace

Molasses: 1 cup 0

Mushrooms: 2 tablespoons 0

Mustard: prepared, 1 teaspoon .... trace

Nectarine: 1 nectarine 1

Noodles: egg noodles, cooked, 1 cup 2

Noodles: chow mein, canned, 1 cup 11

Oil: corn, 1 tablespoon 14
olive, 1 tablespoon 14
peanut, 1 tablespoon 14
safflower, 1 tablespoon 14
soybean, 1 tablespoon 14

Okra: 8 pods .... trace

Olives: green, 4 medium 2

Olives: ripe, 2 large 2

Onions: raw, 1 cup .... trace

Orange: raw, 1 orange .... trace

Orange juice: raw, 1 cup............................ trace

Oysters: raw, meat only, 1 cup 4

Pancake: buckwheat from mix
egg & milk added, 1 pancake......................2

Pancake: plain, home recipe,
1 pancake 2

Peach: raw, 1 peach................................. trace

Peanut butter: 1 tablespoon 8

Peanuts: roasted in oil, 1 ounce...................14

Pears: 1 pear, raw................................... trace

Peas: edible pod, cooked, 1 cup.............. trace

Peas: green, frozen, cooked, 1 cup.......... trace

Pecans: pieces, 1 tablespoon 5

Pepper: green, 1 pepper........................... trace

Pickle: dill, 1 pickle................................ trace

Pickle: sweet, 1 pickle.............................. trace

Pie: apple, 1 piece 18

Pie: creme, 1 piece.......................................23

Pie: pecan, 1 piece.......................................32

Pineapple: raw, 1 cup.............................. trace

Plum: raw, 1 plum .... trace

Popcorn: air popped, 1 cup .... trace

Pork: fresh, chop, broiled, lean only, 2.5
ounces 8 pan fried 11

Pork: shoulder, braised, lean only,
2.4 ounces 8

Pork: sausage, 3 ounces 22

Potato chips: 10 chips 7

Potatoes: baked, 1 potato .... trace

Potatoes: french fried in oil, 10 strips 8

Potatoes: Shake n' Bake® oven cooked,
10 strips 1

Pretzels: made with enriched flour,
2 1/4 inch long, 10 pretzels .... trace

Pudding mix: with whole milk, 1/2 cup 4
with nonfat milk, 1/2 cup 0

Pumpkin: cooked, 1 cup .... trace

Raisins: 1 cup 1

Raspberries: raw, 1 cup 1

Rhubarb: cooked, 1 cup .... trace

Rice: brown, cooked, 1 cup 1

Rice: white, instant, 1 cup 0

Roll: dinner, commercial, 1 roll.................... 2

Roll: Hot dog or hamburger,
commercial, 1 roll............................... 2

Rum: 1 ounce................................ 0

Salad Dressing: Commercial,
Blue cheese,
1 Tablespoon.................................. 8
French, 1 tablespoon......................... 9
Italian, 1 tablespoon......................... 9

Salad Dressing: Fat Free dressings 0

Salad dressing: Mayonnaise, regular,
1 tablespoon.................................. 11

Salad dressing: Mayonnaise, Fat Free,
1 tablespoon.................................. 0

Salami: cooked, 2 ounces...................... 11

Salmon: canned, 3 ounces..................... 5

Salmon: smoked, 3 ounces..................... 8

Salt: 1 cup.................................. 0

Sardines: canned in oil, 3 ounces.............. 9

Sauerkraut: canned, 1 cup.................... trace

Scallops: breaded, 6 scallops 10
steamed, fresh, 1 ounce...................... 1/2

Sherbet: 1 cup.............................. 4

Shortening: 1 tablespoon.............................. 13

Shrimp: canned, 3 ounces 1

Sole: raw, 1 ounce 2

Soup: clam chowder, 1 cup.......................... 7

Soup: cream of mushroom, 1 cup................ 14

Soup: chicken noodle, 1 cup......................... 2

Soup: vegetable beef, 1 cup.......................... 2

Sour cream: (see cream)

Soy Sauce: 1 tablespoon............................... 0

Soy Beans: dry, cooked, drained,
1 cup 10

Soy Product: Miso, 1 cup 13

Soy Product: tofu, piece 2 1/2 by
2 3/4 by 1 inch, 1 piece 5

Spaghetti: no sauce, 1 cup............................ 1

Spaghetti: tomato & cheese sauce,
1 cup 9

Spinach: raw, 1 cup .... trace

Squash: raw, 1 cup...................................... 1

Steak: (see beef)

Strawberries: raw, 1 cup............................. 1

Sugar: granulated, brow or powdered,
1 cup 0

Sunflower Seeds: hulled, 1 ounce 14

Syrup: cane or maple, 1 tablespoon 0

Taco shell: baked, no oil .... trace

Tangerine: 1 tangerine .... trace

Tapioca: pudding, 5 ounces 5

Tatar Sauce: regular, 1 tablespoon 8

Tartar Sauce: with Fat Free
Mayonnaise, 1 Tablespoon 0

Tofu: (see soy product)

Tomatoes: raw, 1 tomato .... trace

Tomato Ketchup: 1 cup .... trace

Tomato juice: 1 cup .... trace

Tomato sauce: 1 cuptrace

Tortilla: corn, uncooked, 1 tortilla .... trace

Tortilla: flour, with shortening, 1 ten inch 3

Tuna: oil pack, 3 ounces 7

Tuna: water pack, 3 ounces 1

Turkey: Ham, 2 ounces 3

Turkey: breast, no skin, 1 ounce 1

Turkey: dark meat, no skin, 1 ounce 1.5

Turnip Greens: raw, 1 cup .... trace

Turnips: cooked, 1 cup .... trace

Veal: cutlet, broiled, 3 ounces 9

Veal: rib, roasted, 3 ounces 14

Venison, 1 oz., lean only, broiled ...less than 1

Vodka: 1 ounce 0

Vinegar: 1 ounce 0

Waffle: home recipe, 1 waffle 13

Waffle: Fat Free, 1 waffle 0

Walnuts: english, 1 cup 74

Water Chestnuts: canned, 1 cup .... trace

Watermelon: 1 cup 1

Whiskey: 1 ounce 0

Wiener: (see frankfurter)

Wine: all kinds, 1 ounce 0

Worcestershire Sauce: 1 tablespoon 0

Yeast: 1 packet .... trace

Yogurt: made with whole milk,
8 ounces 7
Yogurt: nonfat... 0

Yogurt: low fat, plain, 8 ounces 4

Source: United States Department of
Agriculture and individual manufacturers label
information.

Note: For a more complete nutrition analysis
order the U.S. Dept. of Agriculture Home and
Garden Bulletin number 72 titled "Nutritive
Values of Foods". Send $2.75 to:

U.S. Government Book Store
Pueblo, Colorado
81009

ACKNOWLEDGEMENTS AND REFERENCES

"Just No Fat" by Norman Rose sounds like I wrote the whole book. I would like to take full credit, but that would be foolish for me to do so. Several people, more than one professional association, various federal agencies and the University of Kansas Medical Center have all contributed to this book.

My thanks to Warren Walker for his strong editing that made sense out of a lot of varied thoughts in Chapter 3.

Chapter 4 was written by Wallace C. Donohue with permission. Wallace C. Donohue is president and CEO of Creative Health Products, Plymouth, Michigan.

Chapter 6 is essentially a reprint of the National Institute of Health Publication No. 89-2922 entitled, "So You Have High Blood Cholesterol".

Part of the information in Chapter 7, "Eating Out", was obtained from a Human Nutrition Information Service bulletin entitled "Eating Out".

Part of the information in Chapter 9, "Soy Bean and Soy Products - A Rich Source of Protein" was provided by ADM, Archer Daniels Midland Company, Decatur, Illinois and is used with permission.

Part of the information in Chapter 10, Venison, was provided by the New Zealand Farm Ranch Venison Council, Oakland, California, and is used with permission.

Thanks for the information provided in Chapter 11, by the American Bison Association, Denver, Colorado.

Other references include:

The Triglyceride Issue: a view from Framingham, William P. Castelli, M.D. (American Heart Journal 112:432, 1986)

Joint Effects of Serum Triglyceride and LDL Cholesterol and HDL Cholesterol concentration on Coronary Heart Disease Risk in the Helsinki Heart Study, et al. (Circulation 1992; 85:37-45)

Nutritive Value of Foods
USDA Home and Garden Bulletin Number 72

Nutritive Value of American Food
Agriculture Handbook Number 456
Composition of Foods

USDA Agriculture Handbook Number 8

The Effect of Ethanol on Fat Storage in Healthy Subjects by Paulo M. Suter, M.D., M.S., Yves Schutz, Ph.D., M.P.H., and Eric Jequier, M.D., New England Journal of Medicine, Vol. 326, No. 15.

Molly McButter® is a registered trademark of Alberto-Culver Company.

Butter Buds® is a registered trademark of Cumberland Packing Corporation.

Hunt's® is a registered trademark of Hunt-Wesson, Inc.

Grape-nuts® is a registered trademark of Kraft General Foods, Inc.

INDEX OF RECIPES

III. MEAT AND POULTRY

IV. Fish and Shellfish

V. Potatoes, Rice, Pasta & Dried Beans

Potatoes

Rice

VII. Sandwiches, Tacos, Burrito s and Pizza

VIII. Vegetables

X. Desserts

XI. Special Foods